IF I'D OBSERVED ALL THE RULES,

I'D NEVER HAVE GOT ANYWHERE.

– MARILYN MONROE

IF YOU'RE WONDERING WHERE THE

INDEX OR PAGES NUMBERS ARE,

STOP WONDERING.

YOU WON'T NEED THEM.

IF ONLY

It's 2013, and people are utterly convinced that "diets don't work". The most doubtful are those who have never succeeded on one - *and* - those who have never needed one in the first place. So why do we keeping doing them? Well at least in the short term, diets obviously *do* work, a proposition more charming than *James Bond*. But just like 007, they have a dark side: they have a licence to kill... your enjoyment of life.

Even now, some believe the only way to get a good body is to just "eat less and do more exercise". Yes I admit, that *sounds* logical - and deliciously tempting - but we're a complex bunch of apes, and following logic is difficult sometimes. Stuff gets in the way. You know, emotions, bad weather, break-ups, make-ups, families, work, money, hangovers - and of course - what's trending on *Twitter*.

So, what's an ape to do? The smart money - as always - is to turn to science.

It's not perfect, it's not always fast, but it has the biggest ingredient that a happy cake needs. **Proof**. And when it comes to proof, it's in the pudding known as **Intermittent Fasting**. Make no mistake - **it's not the latest fad diet** - and it's not hype presented with a different headline. This is fresh, exciting and brilliant science that works. **It is genuinely amazing.**

Why is Intermittent Fasting so much better than everything before it? Easy. **It has very few rules**. Of course there are some, or you wouldn't need this book. And they might even be tough when you start (the best time for tough). But it's like learning to ride a bike: once you've got the hang of it - **you'll have it forever** - and be able to enjoy the scenery without fear of crashing out.

There is complex science going on behind the simple shrinking, and I'll help you understand what you need. But overall, I'll play to the strengths of *The IF Diet:* **a no-nonsense system that you can see in the palm of your hand, and attack with gusto**. With laser-like focus, humans can do *anything*.

And the easiest way to become laser-like? Just have minimal complication in the first place.

You will *not* need the mental toughness of an SAS soldier, or the brains of a Nobel Prize winning chemist. Girls, you won't need to venture into a gym's free weights area if you don't want, and guys, you won't need to cook weird sounding diet recipes. Actually, **you won't need recipes at all**. Hopefully no one finds those two mentions condescending, because they're often the kind of practical concerns that people have.

Some of you could be wondering why *The IF Diet* doesn't mention ***Alternate Day***, ***5:2*** or ***8 Hour*** on the cover. **Books titled like that focus on just *one* method, and this offers *three*.** The problem with a *one size fits all* diet glove, is that there's a good chance it won't fit *at all*. Guess what? With 3 to pick from - this will glide on perfectly, finger by finger - whatever your job, age, or background. **Congratulate yourself on tripling your routes to success**.

This book is exactly as long as it needs to be - and that's quite short - for a reason. Modern life is spent *dreaming*, *reading*, *waiting* and *debating*, habits which actually do *nothing*. Do "Actions speak louder than words"? Absolutely, but even that *phrase* is words! You see - without action - you're just a big bag of theory. And without successful actions, you're just another diet statistic. Do you want that?

I urge you to read through everything quickly, perhaps in a day, and pick a date - *within 7 days* - on which to start. You're going to pick a date anyway (is it a Monday or a 1st?), so give yourself a moment to prepare mentally, and let the anticipation excite the pants off you. Remember, **this could be your *one life***. And even if it isn't, I bet this one feels important to you *right now*.

The If Diet is in roughly 3 servings. First, I'll zip through the science and give you reasons to be motivated. The best motivation comes from knowing *why* something works. Next, I'll tell you *how* to do it. And finally, for those of you who want to speed things up, I'll cover some of the latest *add-on* techniques.

Intermittent Fasting works brilliantly, but for those who need full speed ahead, this is for them.

And finally, before we get going, here's something to fizzle through your subconscious. Humans appear to vary on the surface - *but under the skin* - we all share a common physiology. That is, *we all work in roughly the same way*. That's what makes medicine a useable science. Modern genes also echo those carried by your prehistoric ancestors. **Whoever who you are - whatever you've tried - *The IF Diet* will work for *you*.**

IF YOU NEED A REMINDER

- diets can work

- you need simplicity

- there are 3 plans in *The IF Diet*

IF BY CHANCE

In 1928, *Doctor Fleming* discovered the antibiotic *Penicillin* because he wasn't keeping his lab in good order. Two years later, American housewife *Mrs Wakefield* was in her kitchen making a chocolate flavored dessert, and ran out of baker's chocolate. She used some broken bits of regular chocolate instead, expecting them to melt and ooze into her dough. They didn't, and *chocolate chip cookies* were born. Unbelievably, *Mrs W* was a dietitian!

The point is, some accidents are happy ones. And that's much the same story with Intermittent Fasting. Long before fitting into skinny jeans became an issue, scientists were mainly concerned with keeping people alive - and if possible - healthy too. A month after World War 2 ended, Chicago scientists *Carlson* & *Hoelzel* published their study on increasing lifespan in rats. They used the *IF* word for the first time.

The truth is, other researchers *had* studied Intermittent Fasting before - but crucially - they *hadn't* spotted the benefits. *Carlson* & *Hoelzel* did. Their rats didn't only live longer, but they were less likely to develop cancer. Even better, rats brought up on Intermittent Fasting grew perfectly. Their leg bones were the same - *or longer* - than regular rats. **And of course, the Intermittent Fasting rats had less body fat**.

Leap forwards to the 20th century, and researchers were still searching for ways to increase lifespan *in humans*. They kept assuming - quite wrongly - that the answer was just to eat less, officially known as "calorie restriction", or "CR". But in humans and monkeys, it didn't work well. Not only that - *dramatic weight loss rarely occurred* - and when it did, it didn't last. **Alas, *constantly* cutting back calories is the #1 diet belief that many cling on to**.

Eventually - and by chance - researchers had their prayers answered by the Islamic holy month of *Ramadan*. During this time, Muslims avoid eating from sunrise until sunset. They then eat regular food. Scientists always believed that this shift of patterns - and gorging without portion control - would lead to health problems.

They predicted that people would get fat and ill. **In fact, it was the opposite**.

They were losing fat, keeping their muscle, reducing their risk of high blood pressure, heart disease and diabetes - and most importantly - **getting all this without eating any special foods**. As you'll see, these are the breakthroughs that other ways of eating - "diets" - don't achieve. The researchers were hooked, and ever since, we've been looking to unlock more secrets. **In 2013, the understanding and use of IF will boom**.

Honestly, it's hard to study Intermittent Fasting. Controlling people in labs is easy, but once they're out, forget it. Because of this, and because those studies are expensive, most research tends to be done on rats (and their cousins, mice). Logically, human studies are best, but I wouldn't ignore all the animal work. Many great discoveries started similarly. Those long legged and slender rodents deserve an extra chunk of cheese for leading the way.

IF YOU NEED A REMINDER

- intermittent fasting was originally designed to increase lifespan

- weight loss and health benefits were then spotted during religious fasting

- human studies now confirm that IF boosts weight loss and general health

IF YOU AVOID ELEPHANTS

Other diets have problems. Each of these problems is an *elephant in the room*, the hugely **OBVIOUS** thing that no one talks about. To be fair, *you* might not see the elephants, but scientists have no excuse. Now, if you understand what these elephants are, you can avoid being crushed by them. As you meet the elephants - *relax* - because I'll explain why you won't be bumping into them on *The IF Diet*.

THE ELEPHANT OF MUSCLE LOSS

As the numbers on your scales go *down*, your happiness goes *up*. But your body isn't just made from "weight". There is *fat weight* and *non-fat weight*. Fat weight = fat. Done. Non-fat weight = muscle, water, organs and bone. **Fat weight is bad and non-fat weight is good**. You need *some* fat weight. If you didn't, you'd be cold, sick, sore, depressed and scary to kids because of your strangely realistic Halloween face.

All other diets will make you lose non-fat weight. Despite the hype, most sudden weight loss isn't "just water". Your body is surprisingly good at hanging onto that. Most sudden weight loss - *and lots of continued weight loss* - includes a loss of *muscle* weight, and *organ* weight. Clearly, shrinking your organs is less than ideal. Why does it happen? It's the body downsizing to cope with a *constant* low calorie recession.

Losing muscle is a disaster. Your nice muscles burn most of your calories. That's why guys burn slightly more calories than girls. As regular diets strip your weight off, they secretly strip your potential to stay slim. With less muscle, it becomes difficult to *keep* weight off.

Intermittent Fasting is the *only* dietary method that will not destroy your muscle tissue. If you want long term fat loss, *The IF Diet* will help guarantee it.

When you ignore away the fancy names and methods, **all diets result in calorie restriction**. And before you say it - *I know* - this has calorie restriction too. But crucially, **Intermittent Fasting doesn't *constantly* reduce calories**. What do I mean by "calorie restriction". Simply eating less than you're "supposed" to. *Supposed* gets put in inverted commas because **estimating calorie needs is highly imprecise**.

Most diets have a calorie restriction of anywhere between 10 and 50%. *Very Low Calorie Diets* - an official medical name for diets of 800 calories or less - are often prescribed for *very* overweight people. At less than 800 cals *day after day*, they can create more problems than they solve. Problems like we've just seen - muscle and organ weight loss - plus gallstones, disruptions to heart rhythm - and of course - putting *lots* of weight back on.

The problems with constantly cutting calories go beyond the physical.

Excess appetite and *giving up completely* are frequent. Let's start, by *giving up*. When dieters have hope, they can do anything. But **losing hope is easy**, especially easy when you're staring at a future involving "being different" all the time. Sticking to constantly low calories *day after day* is BORING! It *will* reduce hope. **Intermittent Fasting - by design - boosts your hope *often***.

With *The IF Diet*, you'll reduce calories *sometimes*, and that's much easier. You'll never go beyond two days in a row of feeling you're "missing out". This is ideal, because if boredom or appetite kicks in - so does will power - driven by the hope of being *just around the corner* from *normal* eating. This is *the* biggest emotional plus with Intermittent Fasting. **By reducing boredom - you increase hope - and this boosts long term success *massively***.

Let's chat about appetite now. If you've ever tried a period of constant calorie restriction - *that's any normal diet* - you will have noticed... *it*. Eventually your appetite *creeps* back - and with so much intensity - that you end up *worse* than when you started.

The science of appetite is outrageously complex and not well understood. It confuses dietitians, doctors, psychologists, sociologists, food makers, market researchers, and even your government.

We believe various hormones and chemicals, including **Leptin**, **Ghrelin**, **Neuropeptide Y**, **Cholecystokinin**, **Serotonin** and **Dopamine** make a difference. Plus the **hypothalamus gland** in general. Oh, and other parts of the brain. You see - or perhaps you don't - that this isn't easy. I say, why not talk about what we *do* know? It's simple: ***constant* calorie restriction eventually causes problems with your appetite, and you get fat again**.

The human body likes to keep things at a nice, even level. Scientists call it **homeostasis**. It's like we have a highly sensitive surveillance team in every part of us. If there's a dramatic change, the body eventually notices it, and steps in to restore order. This system keeps our internal body temperature steady, our blood neither too acidic or too alkaline, and our blood sugar off the rollercoaster. In a nutshell, homeostasis keeps us alive.

Trying to trick this natural status quo isn't easy. It's almost *impossible*. Constant calorie restriction grabs the attention of our internal security guards, and soon enough, they respond by turning up our appetite to the max. They actually turn it up *beyond* our normal maximum, setting the bar so high, that we overeat and get fatter than ever. **Regular diets cause us to eat greater and greater levels of food just to satisfy our appetite**. Drug addiction anyone?

The eagle-eyed amongst you would have noticed the word *almost* before the word *impossible* in the previous paragraph. Why? **Intermittent Fasting *doesn't* boost appetite to a level that's higher than before**. People only eat slightly more on feed days, and this isn't enough to make them fat.

In fact, **people using Intermittent Fasting consistently lose fat and boost all their major health markers**. *The IF Diet* really is a breakthrough.

For many dieters, there is an initial excitement about being *told what to do* within a diet. Some people - believing that a teaspoon of bran might really be magic - are more than happy to follow wacky instructions. But after a few weeks of doing this, the excitement starts to wear off. Limited food choices create 2 problems: **nutrient deficiencies**, and the **embarrassment** of constantly explaining / hiding your weird habits to friends and family.

Explaining what you *can* and *can't* eat isn't enjoyable. After a while, explaining is draining. The ideal diet is one that gives you a good shot at appearing and feeling *normal*. Yes, *The IF Diet* has days or times where you cut back, but that's it.

Intermittent Fasting is unique amongst diets, by giving *you* the choice to pick *your* food. This one fact alone may help you *stay strong* regardless of potential social pressures.

Nutritionally, avoiding any one particular food or food group might have some research to back it up, but real life doesn't care for such precision. Scientists whisper about **Specific Appetite**, a term that describes our subconscious desire to eat foods that correct our dietary deficiencies. This is most obvious in pregnancy, when expectant mothers are known to crave eating *chalk*. They're not weird, *they just need calcium*.

Diets that focus on any particular foods or food group could put you at risk of disease. Nature has developed wonderful mechanisms to help us *self select* foods that prevent it. We have recently discovered hormones and monitoring systems deep in our guts which could help us choose the right amount of protein, the right sources of micronutrients (vitamins and minerals), and even the right intakes of sweet, sour and salty food.

Our best chance of obeying these natural systems, is to get to a healthy body weight, and generally *pick our own food*. That's instead of intentionally restricting food choices on a diet.

Only Intermittent Fasting offers you free choice when it comes to food variety. Some scientists could argue that letting you choose is a risk, or "a gimmick". I respectfully suggest that they're talking *nonsense*. "Nature" is far smarter than "us", at least right now.

Studies show that *higher* **food variety scores** are associated with higher resistance to diseases, higher levels of happiness, and lower levels of obesity. Certain foods - even in nature - may cause problems or benefits when eaten to excess. We don't have a definitive list of what these effects are, or how they interact. Until we do, **use *The IF Diet* to improve your health without the physical and mental hazards of restricted food choice.**

THE ELEPHANT OF RELYING ON EXERCISE

Many diets actually *depend* on exercise as a way of achieving results. Without it, they don't work. Changing your diet is a tough change, and **relying on exercise can cause you to give up entirely**.

Don't get me wrong, exercise is useful for improving many different aspects of health, including mental health. But, it should never be used to make an ineffective diet, effective. **Intermittent Fasting does not _rely_ on exercise to produce results**.

We will explore this in more detail later - but without doubt - exercise _itself_ isn't super effective at improving weight loss. **Exercise can even make weight loss _harder_. Exercise is _not_ essential for weight loss**. I am repeating myself to emphasize the point.

Contrary to yet another myth, modern humans aren't _dramatically_ less active than years ago. We have a dramatically different diet though, and that's where you need to shift your focus.

So there you have it, the elephants of **muscle loss**, **constant calorie restriction**, **limited choice** and **relying on exercise**. Each of those factors are found in every diet outside of Intermittent Fasting. And they create problems which create _more_ problems.

By following *The IF Diet* principles, you will avoid being trampled by this herd of not-so-obvious beasts. **And, you'll give yourself the finest shot at losing weight permanently**.

IF YOU NEED A REMINDER

- normal diets have obvious but rarely mentioned scientific flaws

- they cause muscle loss, boredom, and rely heavily on exercise

- *The IF Diet* is uniquely designed to avoid these problems

IF IT HELPS YOU DETOX

Everyone likes to detox. Get rid of the junk. It's like having a hot shower and getting dressed into fresh clothes (and new socks). Yep, there's definitely that *feel good* factor when you give your body a new start. Most people believe that the most powerful way to detox is to start a classic diet. *"You know, I just want to cut out all the crap"*. Many more assume that juices and smoothies are the way forward.

BREAKING NEWS: the traditional "detox" does not work *at all*.

It will give you a *sense* of doing good - but the real damage is deeper - and there's only one way to fix it. You need a quick biology lesson before I give you the happy news. Your body is built cell by cell - *day by day* - and on a continuous basis. What you eat today, becomes part of you *today*. And tomorrow. And a year from now. Maybe two. Keep reading.

Imagine the nutrients in your diet as *plant food*. If you feed plant food to your favorite Bonsai, it takes a while before you impress *Mr Miyagi*. The old leaves must die off before new ones sprout under the influence of your magical potion. This is the same as your body's cells. Skin takes about 20 days to go from start to finish. Blood cells are born today and reach retirement 90 days later. Muscles take at least 6 months to complete a cycle.

As you live your life, *all* your cells are going through changes. Being born, maturing, dying. Often, some of your cells might have not been "raised" properly. You won't have given them *enough* of the right ingredients, because you followed a limited diet. Perhaps you just ate *too* many chocolate bars. Environmental factors like air pollution, chemicals in the home - *and the unknown* - cause damage too. Sometimes, deep, deep down. That's into our *DNA*.

A regular detox - even a full 7 to 10 days - won't do anything beyond changing surface stuff. Your skin might temporarily clear up. Your eye bags might disappear. Maybe your weight drops a few pounds.

All these changes are minor, and related to you temporarily avoiding inflammatory, allergic and intolerance creating foods.

That's it.

You're washing a car which actually needs a mechanic.

As soon as people finish a detox, they gradually start *adding* back the toxic beauties they enjoyed so much in the first place. Now, I'm certainly not saying that you can't enjoy naughty foods, because you can. But if you want to do a *real* detox, you need something more than turning on the blender and mashing up carrots. **You need to get fully into Intermittent Fasting**.

Now, let's go back to those cells you keep building. Because of our modern world, we often "bring up" lots of our cells *badly*. In fact, we're terrible parents to them sometimes. We bathe them in weird flavored ice creams, fake meats and acidic drinks.

We chuck them copious cookies and chips, and we deprive them of protein. We even take them for walks in traffic choked cities. Our poor cells haven't got a chance.

If you **must** construct something - but don't have the correct materials (a perfect diet) - you have to use alternatives instead. This makes the final product less than ideal. **Try building a footbridge across a canyon with rotten wood**. Guess what. **Your whole body builds footbridges *every* day**. Try building 100,000,000,000 of them without the right materials. How about the brain itself? I doubt even *Steve Jobs* could do that.

Say, you do manage it. What you've built - cheap materials and all - gets damaged further. Air pollution, electromagnetic forces, chemicals, and even too much oxygen sucked in during exercise could *wreck* what you've constructed. Let's add an attack with some *free radicals*, angry little atoms that cause damage *everywhere*. All these things ruin our precious genetic set of building instructions, our **DNA**. Your rickety footbridge is really cracking up.

By now I expect you're slightly disturbed by the *Indiana Jones* storytelling. Relax, Indy's here to rescue you. Actually, it's *Mother Nature*. She invented an amazing process to deal with damage. It's called **Autophagy** - which literally means "self eating". Little garbage guys called **lysosomes**, seek out your sick, dying and random cells, and perform a kind of **internal cleansing**. These cheeky *mad mops* zip around and literally detox you, *inside out.*

If lysosomes find damaged cells, they **eat** 'em up and spit 'em out. *They remove the rotten wood from your footbridge, and burn it.* Lysosomes also look to **repair** entire structures. *They tighten the loosened bolts on your footbridge.* Finally, if lysosomes find unused but useful structures - they break 'em down - and **recycle** the spare parts elsewhere. *They find a boat in the dried up canyon, and use parts of it to replace the rotten wood in your footbridge.*

Autophagy is the ultimate detox process, the real deal.

The humble heroes scientists call **lysosomes** literally deconstruct and reconstruct your body. I assure you, it truly, utterly, and unquestionably blows carrot juicing out of the water! So, what's the deal with mentioning all this? Well, when you're young, autophagy works just fine. As you get older, or more importantly - *as you eat normally* - the process goes wrong.

Regular diets - no matter how "good" the food is - block the *crucial* autophagy process. Simply living a modern life results in *damage build-up*, and our modern way of eating *prevents* that damage from being handled correctly. **Only Intermittent Fasting recreates our natural state, and re-ignites what is meant to be a *continuous process* of damage removal, repair and recycle**.

Around 1900, cancer was rare. A century later, *you* might know someone who has heard the "C" word whispered their way. Some cancers have a strong genetic link - but without a doubt - there are also "non-genetic" factors at play. Your lifestyle and environment take their toll, bit by bit, *year by year*.

If your lysosomes don't take out the trash properly each week - one day - the rats of cancer may come up to street level, and take over permanently.

Cancer, is of course, an extreme example. And, I'm not claiming that Intermittent Fasting will save anyone who already has it. But cancer *is* a process where damage builds up over time, and nature *does* give us autophagy to protect against damage. **For some reason - most likely an evolutionary one - going without food massively activates and boosts the process of autophagy**.

We are living in an era when other diseases are on the rise, and sometimes, we're not sure why. *Alzheimer's Disease* is one of these. Although it's early days, scientists are considering the role of autophagy in this terribly depressing illness. Could it be that our modern way of living - constantly feeding - makes us more vulnerable? Could the lack of regular internal housework be tipping the balance in diseases' favor? Hmmm.

There is no definite answer yet for *Alzheimer's*, but the evidence is building.

Let's lighten the mood now. The human being is an incredible machine. It really is. It's designed for a long life, and it comes with built-in safety mechanisms, monitoring systems, and even an internal repair company. **To keep everything in tip-top shape, all we have to do is keep the repair guys happy by varying our food intake occasionally**.

Intermittent Fasting *definitely and massively increases autophagy*. And thanks to our caveman history, it thrived. In times of little food, lysosomes would race around the body looking for damaged cells, pre-diseased cells, and cells which weren't doing much. It would chop them apart - into their smallest parts - and either burn them for energy, or use them to repair other areas. **Simply, it would perform miracles without any outside help**.

In their quest for finding long life, scientists noticed that those who ate *less*, lived longer and suffered less disease. It's now becoming clear that it's not just about having less itself.

Having *less* means that at some point, you're having good gaps *between* feedings. It's in these gaps that the magic of autophagy occurs. This is undeniable science that I urge you to consider. **It's your design - and your right - to benefit from it,** *right now*.

And *the* most practical way to benefit is to use Intermittent Fasting. **You need a system in place to i-n-t-e-r-r-u-p-t the non-stop way we live**. It's not enough to have longer gaps between lunch and dinner. Sure, that's a nice start, but *Mother Nature* expects more. The garbage guys *can't* do their job if you never give food a rest. This includes those who "eat a perfect diet". **A perfect diet is one that obeys nature's call to "give me a break"**.

IF YOU NEED A REMINDER

- the traditional detox only works temporarily at the surface level

- autophagy is a natural process that detoxes at the cellular level

- to increase autophagy you must practice Intermittent Fasting

IF YOU GET SMARTER

Okay - I know - you're in a hurry to lose weight and don't need any more science lessons! But I want you to know that if you use Intermittent Fasting, there's an unexpected bonus heading your way. *The IF Diet* will make you smarter. And by the way, this is *not* some kind of lame sales pitch! **Intermittent Fasting increases something called BDNF - and that *literally* - makes you smarter**.

BDNF - or *Brain Derived Neurotrophic Factor* for long - is a protein produced in the brain. It's from a family of "growth factors" called **neurotrophins**. This intelligent sounding word describes molecules that increase brain and nervous system growth. The word is from the Greek *neuro* meaning "nerve", and *trophic* meaning "nourishment". I hate complication, so: **BDNF is a chemical that makes your brain and nervous connections grow**.

It exists in other parts of the body too, but BDNF's nervous system role is the most exciting.

We've noticed that in the brains of *Alzheimer's Disease* patients, it's *lower*. We've also seen that in the depressed, it's *lower*. We know that if you reduce levels of BDNF, it's harder to learn *new* things, remember *old* things, and think *critically*. Thinking critically - that's evaluating stuff - is *so* important for becoming a successful human. Crap decisions, crap life.

Without a doubt - whether you're a lab rat or a human - you want high levels of BDNF. *Disrupting it* will make you the rat who never finds the chunk of cheese, or the human who never makes use of their amazing brain. Having optimal levels of BDNF helps your brain "joins the dots" brilliantly - making this wonderful thing called life - a *really* fun school. **The ultimate form of *networking* is when your brain's connections work in perfect harmony**.

Seriously, it's a breakthrough. For years we believed that our brains grew as we did, reaching maturity in the teens, and then slid downhill ever since. Today, we know we *can* boost our brain's *connections*.

Allegedly, better connections between the left and right brain makes women *smarter* than men! It's hard to define "intelligence" - but this *is* certain - **by enhancing your brain's connections, your potential for intelligence *is* higher**.

Hopefully the thought of increasing your BDNF is almost as exciting as downsizing your *Levis*. And, there is an easy way to make your brain an all-singing, all-dancing, zinging super-computer. Use Intermittent Fasting. **When you give your body a break from food, you give your brain a break too**. Scientists are now starting to understand how the process of *temporarily going without* makes your brain **dramatically** boost its own effectiveness.

It all makes complete evolutionary sense. If your brain senses that you can't get food, it helps you out. Well, it's helping itself out. It raises BDNF levels, and you build new connections. Your newly enhanced intellect makes you a better hunter. You remember where that meaty bison was hanging out. You build better tools.

You learn how to use them better. And, you think carefully before chewing on that strange mushroom that looks *wrong*.

The net result is that the brain lives to fight another day, and you become a better provider overall. Now the smartest way to get even smarter, isn't to permanently reduce calories, as seen in normal diets. That practice of *constant restriction* is both miserable, and it misses the evolutionary point. **You simply need to have times where food *isn't* coming in**. You need gaps. *The IF Diet* plans give you the gaps.

A LITTLE BIT OF WHAT YOU DON'T FANCY

Yet again, the Greeks have coined a word for a process that explain stuff. **Hormesis**. It roughly means "rapid motion". I like to think they just meant "boost". Hormesis is the principle by which a small dose of something - *a stress* - causes the body to adapt positively against it. This principle allowed us to vaccinate people against disease.

It happens when you exercise correctly. It also happens when you diet correctly, using Intermittent Fasting.

A small amount of stress acts like a boost, but too much is too bad. When you wear a good pair of shoes, a tiny amount of rubbing makes your skin tougher in that area. Those shoes will remain comfortable, because your feet have adapted. Wear a *nasty* pair of shoes - and keep wearing them despite the pain - and you'll tear into your skin. Ouch. A little dose is good, too much is too bad. **You could say that the optimal dose, is an *intermittent* dose**.

ALL, NONE, OR SOME

If you stress your brain all the time - *by never eating* - you'll die. If you stress your brain none of the time - *by always eating* - it will never have a reason to improve itself. Finally, if you stress it some of the time - *by Intermittently Fasting* - it will adapt by growing. Hormesis works when you apply the right kind of stress, in the right kind of dosage.

Could it be summed up a bit easier? **It's just about having *gaps*.**

Modern diets - regardless of what's in them - don't give you gaps. **Without gaps, your brain is without reasons to boost BDNF**. I know that I'm repeating myself, both here and throughout the book, but it's important to hammer home the message. **Our modern way of eating doesn't work**. It makes us fatter. Dumber. Sicker. It even makes us sadder. **Only Intermittent Fasting gives us a safe, free and reliable boost**.

IF YOU NEED A REMINDER

- we make BDNF, a chemical that helps learning, memory and thinking

- other diets cause BDNF to drop, which then drops your mental performance

- intermittent fasting reliably raises BDNF to help enhance your mental development

IF I CAN CHOOSE

You've made it past the science. Well, most! There are many ways to make Intermittent Fasting work. We will focus on three. With a bit of research - especially online - you'll find lots more. The problem is, they have no scientific or long-term practical basis. That's okay if you're happy to be a walking human experiment - or go for short-term success - but why bother? Until we find smarter ways, stick to what works brilliantly time after time.

All three methods work in a scientific sense. You will bump into people, either physically or online, who will swear that only one of them is useful. They're wrong. If you were living in a supervised laboratory - *over time* - the plans could organize themselves into order of "best to worst". But real life isn't a lab. **What's "best" is what works for you.** What's "worst" are all the methods that are supposed to work, but don't.

Coming up are the quick summaries of the plans.

If you skim through them, you'll instinctively get a feeling for which one suits you, at least in theory. And, if you're in a hurry, skip to the following chapters that explain your chosen method in more detail. Listen up: you don't have to stick to one plan all the time. Jobs change, people change, the world changes. **You are allowed to change.**

THIRDER PLAN

• Eat normally, but do it within an 8 hour time gap

This is a fantastic intro to Intermittent Fasting. It's simple, and fits neatly into many people's schedules. You will consume all of your calories in a third of your 24 hour day. For example, you might choose to eat between 1pm and 9pm. For the remaining two thirds of the day, that would be from 9pm to 1pm the next day, you'll not be eating. And of course, for some of that time - hopefully a decent chunk of that time - you'll be asleep.

This plan isn't designed to make you cram extra food into a relatively short period. And happily, most people don't end up doing that once they've adjusted. It's simply a way of bringing back some order into the modern habit of non-stop munching. **You can arrange the 8 hour eating time to suit your life**. Hate skipping breakfast? Don't do it then. Hate skipping dinner? Don't do that either. It's very flexible, and easy to slot into.

SWITCHER PLAN

- **eat normally one day - eat 500 to 600 calories the day after - and repeat**

This is what many people know as "alternate day fasting". Perhaps the use of the word *fasting* is slightly unfair, because on the alternate days, you will get to eat something. And you'll always have access to drinks. In a biological sense, this plan closely resembles how we would have lived thousands of years ago. This makes it highly effective, in terms of pure results.

The body quickly learns how to make the best use of food, and adapts quickly.

In a psychological sense - this plan may *sound* inflexible - because many people don't like an every-other-day type of order. But for some, this weakness is actually a strength. They actually like the burst of effort *every so often*, and find it's practically the only way to stick at something. In our modern world of unstructured working habits, this plan might suit certain occupations particularly well.

WEEKENDER PLAN

• Eat normally 5 days a week - and on the other 2 days - eat 500 to 600 calories per day

I've called this *Weekender* because it makes it easier to grasp this as a two days in-a-row method. **You don't have to do it on weekends at all** (of course some hard working folk claim they "never get weekends"!). You just need to pick any couple of back-to-back days where you can apply it.

Two days per week is a useful amount of time from a scientific sense, and it's also useful in a practical sense.

Scientifically, most of the health and weight loss benefits from Intermittent Fasting occur quickly (24 to 48 hours), then settle down. Psychologically, motivation determines a *massive* part of your success, and that's relatively easy to keep going for a couple of days. This plan is like heading to the office on Monday and Tuesday, and then having Wednesday to Sunday at home. Sound tempting? This could be the plan for you.

SEE THE FISH CLEARLY

In life, lots of your fears will be exaggerated. **If you stare *through* a fishing bowl, you'll see a big fish. If you stand *above* the bowl and look down into it, you'll see that fish is tiny**. This diet isn't difficult. In the grand scheme of things, it's easy. And it's *much* easier than going through life not having the body, health and mind that you desire.

There's enough choice within these pages to help you get that. **If you want it, come and get it**.

IF YOU NEED A REMINDER

- you use Intermittent Fasting by varying food intake

- no system is perfect apart from what's perfect for you

- there are *Thirder*, *Switcher* and *Weekender* plans to choose from

IF I GO THIRDS

• **Eat normally, but do it within an 8 hour time gap**

Probably the most powerful thing about Intermittent Fasting, is how it teaches your body to *rely on itself* from time to time. That *one* change is extremely influential. Unfortunately, most humans *rely on food* way too much. Lucky for you, you're not most humans. The **Thirder** plan is a great way to get your body purring in sync with nature's design, and do it every day. You will eat "normally", but do it within an 8 hour time slot.

8 hours *is* a long time. Assuming you have normal sleep patterns, it's about half the time you're awake. Food is fantastic, but you still don't need more than 50% of your eyes-open life to stare at the stuff. What's useful with this plan, is a built-in flexibility that fits around the life you already enjoy. With *Thirder*, you're simply *shifting* your feeding patterns, and there are 3 ways to customize it.

For example **Eating between 3pm and 11pm**

Lots of people prefer to eat later at night. Are you one? Perhaps you like to chew while watching evening television, and get a double hit of the feel-good brain chemical *dopamine*. Or maybe you prefer to share calories and conversation, another dopamine double whammy. Do you think I'm about to tell you it's bad for you? Well, I'm not. Because it isn't. Research has tried to find a problem with eating late, and it's come up with zilch.

Of course, if you eat all day and *continue* to eat at night, you could accuse eating late of pushing your body past its needs. But the act of eating your food later - *in itself* - doesn't affect your chances of being slim. This is good news, and not just for those who simply can't watch a movie without munching. If your winters are dark, late food can be very comforting. Anthropologists believe this late night preference could reflect our fireside cave habits.

There is one piece of take home advice regarding late night eating. **Make sure there is at least 60 minutes from your last mouthful, to the time you think you'll fall asleep**. This is important to maximize **growth hormone** output. Growth hormone repairs your entire body. Very high blood sugar makes it difficult to release, and most of the release normally happens in the first few hours of sleep. Leaving a small gap before then is sensible.

Also, a full stomach - either from solids or liquid - could be uncomfortable and keep you awake. If you're not sleeping deeply or have a broken sleep, you won't produce the optimal *amount* of growth hormone. For some, there's a fine line between going to bed hungry, and going to bed stuffed. With a bit of practice, you can find the balance. Of course, social events play havoc with food timing sometimes. Just do the best you can.

Many have a fear - and a belief - that missing out on breakfast is dangerous. **It isn't**. Research confirms that in *some*, skipping breakfast leads to overeating in other meals. This has never been shown in **Intermittent Fasting**. Besides - with 8 hours to feed yourself - you won't suffer any negative effect. Remember, Intermittent Fasting works well by **using your own fuel**, and delaying your first meal does *exactly* that.

During the night - your body continues to function - carrying out repairs and keeping you dreaming. By morning, your blood sugar will be low. It never reaches zero, so you *will* have energy to go about your day. Elite Kenyan distance athletes start theirs via an hour's run *without food*. The point isn't "but I'm not an elite Kenyan distance athlete". The point is, *ultra* **high levels of human activity** *are* **possible without breakfast**.

The *Ramadan* research shows that regular people also do fine without breakfast. Remember - these are your fellow humans, not rats - and many of them are going without *any* liquid. You *will* get liquid, which makes a big difference. In the studies, health markers improve constantly from day 1 to day 30. It's quite interesting to note that within Islam, there are very few excuses for not "keeping the fast", with only the truly sick being exempted.

If you struggle in the beginning, remember that this can simply be your body going through a *phase* of adjustment. There is a good chance that you may have had slightly poor blood sugar control **before** you started *The IF Diet*, and missing your *Cheerios* simply highlighted it. **A healthy human should not suffer - at all - from *temporary* food deprivation**. Happily, one week of this plan is enough to make you adapt and *thrive* on it. Be patient.

THE DAY SHIFT

For example **Eating between 12pm and 8pm**

You could be someone who has no preference for eating early or late. Maybe your work schedule means that eating in the "middle" portion of the day is a social priority. If that's you, this particular variety of the *Thirder* plan will suit. From a physical perspective, it's well balanced. **Moving around on empty** in the morning burns fat fast, while **sleeping on empty** guarantees a late night surge in growth hormone production.

Unlike *The Night Shift* you won't have long to wait before you eat something. A small 4 or 5 hour gap is extremely doable. For many, this is an optimal amount. Regardless of your occupation, simply being awake requires energy, and going without food for this mini chunk of time will force your body to **tap into fat**. And then, you *will* "break" your "fast" around the traditional time for lunch, or slightly earlier.

With the timings of food in our example - *12pm to 8pm* - there's still time to eat comfortably *after* a typical day's work. The few hours spare after that also means that your blood sugar gets time to drop before you drop off to la-la land. This guarantees a solid *burst* of growth hormone while sleeping. **Growth hormone arrives in "waves" throughout the night, and the most powerful of these is within the first 90 minutes of shut-eye**.

For many people who use the *Thirder* plans, *The Day Shift* is perhaps the most practical. It requires a small sacrifice at the beginning and end of each day, in exchange for a big improvement. Of all the three variations within *Thirder*, this allows you to get benefits with minimal disruption to your regular routine. Combined with the well-judged use of liquids (coming up soon), it's highly effective.

THE MORNING SHIFT

For example **Eating between 9am and 5pm**

Some people have made their minds up: they *absolutely* can't function without a particular meal. Hand on heart, that's nonsense. **All healthy humans can miss a meal, or two**. If you can't, you have simply formed strong *habits*. Habits can be psychological to start with, and *physiological* soon after. Relax, I'm not here to *demand* change. I love you just the way you are. Just like your parents who once sent you to bed without your dinner!

The early part of this plan should be fine, as you're getting to eat normally. It's the latter part that some don't bargain for. Remember - if you're *choosing* an easy start - you're choosing a slightly harder finish. Harder, but not impossible.

During the low carb craze of the late 1990s, people were regularly "cutting out carbs" after a certain time each evening. Many of these dieters did well for a while, before eventually junking out a few months later.

In their case, it was the specific *low carb* advice that set them up for disaster. Intermittent Fasting does not single out any particular food or food group, so it's unlikely that you'll suffer cravings in the evening. The key is to **eat a balance of foods within your 8 hour feeding gap**. Do *not* limit yourself to any particular food or style of eating during this time. **The fact that you're fasting afterwards is enough**. Eat instinctively.

So there you have it, another choice within a choice. If you're going to do the *Thirder* plan, you may need to experiment with a few different time slots before sticking with it. The time of the examples used above are *just examples*. I don't know how your life works on a daily basis, so only you will be able to *fine tune* things. **Whichever option you choose, you should start to feel and see changes within 7 to 10 days**.

In terms of *what to eat*, it's easy: **eat normally within the 8 hours**. At the end of the book, there are some extra thoughts about food, and you could use these to help you out. But you don't *have* to. There are many ways to improve a diet's *quality*. **The intention of *Thirder* is to improve your entire diet *structure***. This itself will help you lose weight, and improve a wide variety of general health markers.

CHANGING SHIFTS

On a couple of days per week - and I mean just *two* days - you can change the position of your 8 hour feeding period. This is handy for those who have a few days where eating at different times makes more sense. Perhaps these are days off from work, or simply days where something social is happening, you need to make that a priority. These couple of days can feel like a refreshing release of steam.

I would *definitely* limit these changes to twice per week at most. Why? If you change *all the time*, there will be an immense temptation to slip back into normal eating, *all the time*. Before you know it, *The Night Shift* will run into *The Morning Shift*, and you'll soon just be eating around the clock. That's not Intermittent Fasting. That's constant feeding! Cut yourself some slack a couple of days per week, and leave it at that.

You don't need to let any of this section scare or confuse you. Hey, it's just **eating normally, but within an 8 hour time gap**. I know this sounds strange now, but just setting a date, and giving it a go one day *can* be fun. If *Thirder* really doesn't sound like it's for you, read on. The next plan, *Switcher* is quite different. And even if that doesn't suit you - there's more reading material - handily called, *Weekender*.

IF YOU NEED A REMINDER

- the *Thirder* plan is eating normally but within an 8 hour time period

- you can place these 8 hours to cover your mornings, days, or nights

- up to twice a week you can shift from one variation to another

IF I SWITCH

• **Eat normally one day - eat 500 to 600 calories the day after - and repeat**

This plan is the classic "alternate day" style commonly associated with Intermittent Fasting. Having said that, early versions alternated normal eating with days of *zero* calories. We're *not* going for zero. **This style of Intermittent Fasting works best if you eat no more than about 25% of your regular calories**. Now, we could attempt to calculate exactly what 25% means for you, but precision and complication are neither interesting or necessary.

Some researchers suggest a 500 calorie daily limit for women, and 600 for men. But it's the age of equality, and I like simple. **Whether you're male or female, aim to eat *between* 500 and 600 calories on fast days**. Women are no longer kept down souls who stay at home knitting.

Modern women have similar activity levels to modern guys, and they're often similarly sized. Besides, I wouldn't want to start any inter-gender calorie gloating!

So, we're covering the basics quickly. **One day you eat "normally" - whatever that means for you - and on the next day you do a modified fast, by eating 500 to 600 calories**. Now, those 500 to 600 calories are going to feel very valuable to you. You will *savor* them. Is there any way to make them more pleasurable? Yes there is. These easy to follow tips will help you do that.

DIVIDE AND CONQUER

The first thing you can try, is splitting your calories into smaller parts. I mean, *small meals*. How many? **A maximum of two meals in general - but for the first week - you can use three**. This gives your body *and* mind a chance to adapt. The brilliance of Intermittent Fasting is its laid back approach to a complex problem.

My goal is to always simplify that further, by helping you **set up the rules to win**. Always make change *smooth*.

So - if you need to - **for the first week, divide 600 calories into three meals**. You *don't* have to be precise, and hit 200 / 200 / 200. It's possible for a day or so, but highly irritating after that. More importantly, it's not necessary. **When your body is on a modified fast (I say "modified" because it's not a true *zero* calorie "fast"), it will extract energy and nutrients whatever way you present them**.

For the cheeky rebels, please don't think about dividing everything into *more than* 3 meals. This could be tempting, especially if you're planning on eating 6 of your favorite 100 calorie chocolate bars! And believe it or not, I've nothing against chocolate. **Eating more frequently than three times per day - *even at less than 600 calories in total* - could ignite hormonal systems that keep you holding fat**.

It's in the gaps *between* eating where the magic happens. Food stimulates **insulin**, a hormone that takes whatever's floating in your blood, and locks it up in cells. It may lock carbs into muscles as energy reserves - or send them into fat cells - where they *become* fat. **Insulin does many things - *sometimes good* - but on fast days, we want it low**. When the insulin dragon sleeps, fat-busting beauties like growth hormone come out and make you slim.

After a week, have your 600 calories spread over two meals *maximum*.

Although this sounds restrictive, it now means that each meal can be more substantial. You know, like a regular meal. **I do not suggest going down to one meal**. Why? It's mentally tougher with just one opportunity to eat. Plus, it's harder socially. Strangely, **eating once could reduce the *variety* of foods you get, compared to two feeds**. You'd eat *more* of *fewer* foods.

Now, the question often comes up, "When should I eat these meals?". The happy answer is **it doesn't seem to make a difference *when* you eat**. Again, this is due to you becoming extremely *efficient* at dealing with food. I'd still avoid eating *just* before sleep. Otherwise you'll reduce the natural surge of growth hormone that comes with drifting off. I fully appreciate the need for a later meal if that's your preference, just not *too* late.

Certainly for practical reasons, it's nice to separate the 600 calories up to suit whatever kind of lifestyle you have. Within a very short period, you will discover when it's perfect for you. Unlike *Thirder*, you have no time restrictions. It's perfectly acceptable to have a morning and evening meal on one day, and say, an afternoon and evening one on the next.

Mixing it up randomly will not reduce results, assuming you duck under 600 calories on fast days.

I am *not* going to give you specific dietary guidelines in this section. That would defeat *The IF Diet* spirit. But, I would like to give you one tip that seems to work for everyone. **Get more protein**. The word *protein* is from the Greek meaning "of first importance". Various food factors increase what scientists call **satiety**, or what most people call *fullness*. Actually, it's more **the feeling of fullness mixed with happiness**.

If you can increase satiety, you can increase your chance of sticking to the plan. Simply, **protein seems to manage our hunger better**. Fiber increases satiety, by causing a gloopy mess within the stomach. You can read more about it later. Fat increases it too, but at 9 cals a gram - and occupying not much space in your stomach - it's not as good as protein. Protein - at 4 cals a gram and requiring more stomach space - satisfies the brain *brilliantly*.

Now as I said, I'm not going to give you complex advice, or gram by gram food tables to stare at.

All of that increases anxiety towards food. I only suggest being more *mindful* of protein. If you're struggling to get by with 600 calories on fast days, **don't give up without *upping* your protein**. Most scientists still argue about *why* protein works - but importantly - all scientists agree that it *does* work.

Okay, so you at least want some sources of protein. Well, to get you started, think meat. Obvious, I know. Meat - by definition - is protein. It will have some fat, and minimal carbs. I'm not going to reel off a list of meats, apart from reminding you that fish is meat too. Surprisingly, many people consider themselves vegetarians if they "only" eat fish! And what happens if you *are* a vegetarian?

You should still be *mindful* of protein. Vegetarians are not magically different to meat eaters in terms of general health. You can still be very unhealthy as a vegetarian, so it's important that you approach this book with equal effort. Vegetarian sources of protein are fewer, and heavily concentrated around soy based products. Beans, nuts, yogurts, quinoa, cheese and eggs (for those who eat them) are also things to help you out.

Many dieters are obsessed with fatty foods, as in, they do whatever they can to avoid them. In a general sense, **fat in food is not solely responsible for making people gain *body* fat**. In fact, two fats - *Omega 3* & *6* - are beneficial for heart, brain, development (pregnancy) and cell health. It's an uphill struggle trying to convince dieters that fat isn't evil, so this is why I'm now going to answer a question you're likely to ask.

Will high fat foods on *600 calorie days* reduce the results from Intermittent Fasting? **No**. At times of low calorie intake, your body takes what it can. This is an entirely logical reaction. Now, I answered that question to make the "rules" easier for you to follow. I'm *not* recommending that you eat *more* or even *less* fat.

Apart from being mindful of protein, **I want *you* to enjoy the *freedom* of picking *your* 600 calories**. *Don't* be scared.

On non-fasting days, the advice is simple again: *eat normally*. You'll tend to eat *slightly* more on normal days, compared to if you hadn't fasted the day before. Let me explain with some rough numbers. On fast days, you eat about 25% of your normal calories. On feed days, you will probably eat around 110% of your normal calories (as in a *bit* more than normal). In other words, **over two days you eat much less than normal**. No? Try this:

Average day before *The IF Diet* = 2000 calories

You start *The IF Diet* Switcher plan

Fast day = 600 calories

Feed day = 2200 calories

Average *Switcher* intake = 1400 calories (600 + 2200 = 2800, then divide by 2 days)

You can see the benefits already. **Cutting back on one day doesn't cause a massive overcompensation on the next**. Overall, you will manage to cut down and save *lots* of calories. This itself will cause weight loss. But **the benefits of the 600 cal days themselves go beyond mere calorie mathematics**. Because of the low food intake, **insulin** drops low too. **When insulin is low - *growth hormone is high* - and fat burning takes place *rapidly*.**

THE FORTUNE 600

If you struggle to get under 600 calories on fast days, *don't just give up*. If you've come from 6000 calories per day before that, *of course* it will be hard to start with. When Intermittent Fasting has been studied, it usually gets studied within labs, where kind scientists keep a close eye on everything and everyone. I admit - in that situation - it's a lot easier to keep motivated. But even without those men in white coats, **you can do this**.

You need to become your own scientist.

I mean it. *You* need to find ways of getting under 600. Try *gradually* lowering your daily calorie intake. For example, you begin with a few every-other-day attempts at **1500**. Then you try **1200** on the next attempt. Maybe it takes two weeks of alternate days to handle that. So what! ***You* make the best rules**. Then you hit **900**. By now, the body will help *you*. **Before you know it, 600 is a breeze**.

Don't punish yourself if you creep over 600 - or in the case of what we just discussed - your temporary upper limit. It's about *sweet-talking* your body back to a more efficient place. Beating it over the head isn't necessary. One of *the* most powerful ways to get through things, is having the support of someone who cares about you. Ideally, they do *The IF Diet* with you. **Teamwork really achieves miracles**.

Are you still confused by all of this? Don't be. It's simple. **Eat normally today - then tomorrow - try getting by with 600 calories, spread over a couple of mini meals**. Job done. And after you do that, just repeat.

So - if after all this you're *still* not happy - smile, because it's time for the *Weekender* plan. It uses many of the same principles here, and just arranges them in a different way.

IF YOU NEED A REMINDER

- the *Switcher* plan is eat normally one day, 600 calories the next, and repeat

- you can divide your 600 calorie days into 2 meals (or 3 in the first week)

- the meals can be eaten *when* you like, and can be made from *what* you like

IF I LOVE WEEKENDS

• Eat normally 5 days a week - and on the other 2
days - eat 500 to 600 calories per day

Straight off, this *isn't* about weekends. Sorry 'bout
that. In fact, most people wouldn't like to spend
their most relaxing days eating *less*. The *Weekender*
plan is really about doing two back-to-back lower cal
days, and doing what you want on the next 5.
**Weekender is designed for people who prefer
a burst of effort, and then normality for the
majority of their time**. **The two days in-a-
row can be *any* two days in-a-row**.

This plan also suits people who have a generally
"fixed" lifestyle. If you know roughly where you'll
be on certain days of the week, or know which days
are really important to you, *Weekender* could be ideal.
**The certainty of knowing *what* will happen
when, may reassure you**. And feeling reassured
is *extremely* useful if you have to psych yourself up for
those 600 calorie days. The *Switcher* plan might not
fit personalities who need that.

So, how does this **2 days on / 5 days off** still work? The maths whizzes amongst you will have realized that the figures don't add up like in *Switcher*. You're correct. It's difficult to generate exact figures anyway - but *Weekender* works well - despite not causing the same overall calorie loss of *Switcher*. How? Because **Weekender strongly improves your body's food handling efficiency even when you're *off***.

ALL NIGHT LONG

Many of the benefits with Intermittent Fasting happen within 24 hours. That's what makes *Thirder* and *Switcher* effective. But beyond 24 hours, you can create an effect that lasts for *longer*. And this is what happens on *Weekender*.

Two consecutive low calorie days cause a dramatic shift in how your body deals with food.

When you return to "normal" eating, the benefits of this shift *linger*. And, they linger *just* enough to see you through another 5 days.

THE PERFECT COUPLE

Why *two* days? We're used to handling a couple of days of *something*. A couple of days detox, *easy*. A couple of days staying up late, *easy*. A couple of days forgetting work, really *easy!* **Two days in a row - *psychologically* - is an easy time period to focus on**. Going from 1 to 2 days is a 100% increase. That means with a bit more mental effort - *an extra day's push* - you get a doubling of the physical effect. Actually, it's more than double.

But what about putting in *another* day's effort, and go from 2 to 3 days in a row? That's a 50% increase. 3 to 4 days? A 33% increase. Some might scoff at these calculations, but that's roughly how your body responds. With more days in a row, you get an ever smaller bang for your buck. I mean, it's just not worth it. Why? Your body loves *homeostasis*.

It's Greek for "standing still". It will slowly find ways to *do nothing* if you stress it too much.

It can do this by making you tired. It can also drop your hormones and body temperature to make you "save calories". It could even allow you to get ill - *unintentionally* - because of a depleted immune system. In a nutshell, **fasting two days in-a-row is best**. It's a big rock splashing in a lake, creating *ripples* that keep coming for a while. Much better than dropping an asteroid down and destroying the lake entirely.

The principles of **what to eat** and **when to eat** are the same as *Switcher*. That is, **eat normally, and eat when it suits you best**. Ideally - **spread the 600 cals over 2 meals** - but use 3 during the first week if you need them. Time the meals to suit whatever your schedule requires, and that's about it. **With two low cal days in-a-row, your body will become *extremely* efficient at handling food**. The ripple of change will bathe you kindly for days.

The first of those 5 days is the time where you'll eat *slightly* more than normal. Don't panic. **This is to be expected**. By the way - I'm not *telling* you to eat more - I'm saying it might happen. By the second of those 5 days, you'll probably be close to "normal", whatever that is for you. Again, **don't panic if you feel you're overeating**. As weeks go by, you'll find that the whole 5 days become "normal" and quite controlled.

DOUBLE DETOX

If you use *Weekender*, you may find that you get withdrawal symptoms over the two days. And that's literally because you're behaving differently for two days in-a-row. On the other plans, because there's never two days in-a-row, withdrawal symptoms rarely occur. You could be wondering *what* "withdrawal symptoms" I keep talking about. Generally, I'm talking **caffeine** (which you can still have by the way), but it could be other things.

In our food and drink supply, there are many nutrients and unknowns which sneakily create a state of dependence.

You may - *without realizing* - gravitate towards eating and drinking these. I'm not saying they're bad. It could be your body directing you towards what it actually *needs*. I'm saying that on 600 calorie fast days, you might not get enough of what you're withdrawing from. You might get withdrawal symptoms like a **headache** or **rash**.

As with *Switcher*, take your time to get used to it. Don't think that one failed attempt at two days in-a-row means "give up" time. No, no, no. Give *it* time. Give *you* time. Of course, you might have to wait 5 days for your next attempt, but that's great. You can psych yourself up, plan your *dream* 600 calories! This entire process is about setting up *simple* rules to help you win.

Do everything with a smile, because it's fun.

IF YOU NEED A REMINDER

- the *Weekender* plan is 600 cals for two days in-a-row, followed by 5 normal days

- back-to-back fast days boost how your body handles food throughout the week

- two days in-a-row is easy to focus on and works well in those with fixed schedules

IF I NEED A DRINK

Some of the earliest human fasting science came from studying Muslims during the holy month of *Ramadan*. Although researchers witnessed many positive health changes, they also noticed tiredness in some, and blamed it on the reduction in food. In fact, this fatigue was almost always due to dehydration. Under Islamic rules - from sunrise to sunset - nourishment must not pass the lips, and that includes *water*.

We now understand that being dehydrated is bad for humans. Holy fasting is there to acknowledge the less fortunate members of society, and in that respect, it succeeds. But if you're using Intermittent Fasting to lose weight and improve your general health, **you must be normally hydrated.**

And that brings me neatly to the first thing you're allowed to consume when fasting.

Let's kill the cliché. **There is no magic "8 glasses per day" recommendation**. And, there is no complex formula for you to remember. In fact - *there is* - but *Mother Nature* computed it for you a long time ago. It's called **thirst**. Contrary to urban and scientific myth, **thirst *is* a great indicator of when you need to hydrate**. It's not "too late" once you feel thirsty. It's strange to think that scientists ever doubted her accuracy.

When it comes to speed, **plain water is absorbed faster than any other source**. Always was and always will be, regardless of what drink manufacturers say. By the way, **being *over* hydrated has no benefits**. If you have more water than you need, your kidneys will navigate you to the nearest toilet. As mentioned a few moments ago, it's being *de* hydrated that should concern a dieter - or in fact - any human (or pet).

Our smallest parts - *our cells* - are much like us.

If they're really dry, they get tired and don't do a good job. This applies to all cells, regardless *of* their job. Dehydrated muscle cells will make you weak. Dehydrated brain cells will turn your imagination to mud. Dehydrated skin cells won't protect you against the elements. You get the picture. **Dehydration for someone using Intermittent Fasting would mean less than maximum results**.

During fasting periods - assuming you're normally hydrated - you'll produce *especially* large releases of growth hormone. Growth hormone is crucial in both men and women. It's often called the master hormone. The more you make, the more you slim. Exercise is another booster of growth hormone, and studies show that dehydration blocks that boost too. **If you're thirsty, just grab some water**. What about other drinks?

GREEN TEA DURING FASTING

Green tea - which is actually the same plant as black tea - is a pleasant, almost calorie-free drink.

I say "pleasant", because frankly, many people *hate* it! If you happen to like it - and if you take it without sugar or milk - you're in for a "pleasant surprise". **Green tea has been shown to slightly increase your metabolic rate** (the *speed* at which you burn calories). It could also reduce appetite.

How does it manage this? Well, in the case of *green* tea, it's not the caffeine content, because there isn't much. Green tea's main researched component - *Epigallocatechin Gallate* (EGCG) - increases nervous system hormones, including adrenaline. **This increases heat production - and heat has to be paid for - by calories**. There are other benefits related to glugging down EGCG, but the science is mind-blowing and *not* worthy of our time.

Green tea does seem to reduce appetite slightly. Again, the mechanisms are complex, and a full explanation would need a book in itself. Possible theories include *the stimulation of gut hormones* which convince the brain that fullness has arrived. Some research - both for the metabolic and appetite effects - have demonstrated boosts as small as 2%.

That may sound ridiculously small - *but over time* - every little percent adds up.

In terms of effective doses, **you would need to make green tea a regular tipple**. 4 cups per day is optimal. Green tea's chemicals are surprisingly resistant to heat damage, so brewing your tea for 3 minutes or more is safe *and* beneficial (you can still drink it cold). I suggest that you **don't** buy green tea *extract* pills or supplements. Wherever possible, stick close to nature. Nature's "brand" is always the most absorbed.

COFFEE DURING FASTING

If you like coffee, this will make you like it more. **Black coffee** is a rich source of **caffeine**. In plants, caffeine acts as an insecticide to scare off insects. In humans, it's a powerful *Central Nervous System* stimulant that scares off body fat (okay, not literally!). **It helps unlock stored body fat into the blood stream, where you can begin to burn it. And, it increases heat production, which leads to calorie loss**.

Caffeine does have downsides. It's a mild *diuretic*, which means it tells your kidneys to get rid of spare body water. We now think that the water part of coffee balances out the caffeine induced *run-to-the-bathroom* part. If you're in any doubt, just **follow your thirst**. The main problem with caffeine - in *some* people - is that the nervous system stimulation causes a disruption in sleep patterns.

Throughout the day, a chemical called **adenosine** normally builds up, hour by hour. Adenosine *dampens* down brain activity, eventually allowing us to drift off. Caffeine causes mischief - because it *looks* like adenosine - and jumps into the places where adenosine normally builds up. With the spaces blocked - adenosine can't get in to tell your brain "dim the lights" - and we stay... *un* sleepy.

In some, this effect doesn't seem to be strong. One person could drink gallons of coffee and sleep like a log, while another might feel perky just sniffing a *Starbucks* napkin. Obviously, you know who you are. Specific milligram amounts of caffeine are meaningless in everyday life, so I'll state the obvious:

If you can drink *black coffee*, and don't feel it affects your sleep, drink some when fasting.

OTHER LIQUIDS DURING FASTING / GUM

We live in a calorie conscious culture, and big business has responded by designing foods and drinks that contain nothing more than *taste*. They do this with artificial sweeteners, flavorings and colors. Colors affect how we *think* something will taste. In the last few years, it's the sweeteners who have come under fire as a potential health hazard. I don't like messing with nature - but the truth is - research is struggling to find their danger in humans.

Some research shows sweeteners to be the *Oscar* winning actors of the taste world. They are great at *pretending* to be full of calories, when they generally have less than 1. Because of this, there are scientists who believe sweeteners could interfere with our long-term eating habits. Specifically, they believe sweeteners could cause us to *overeat*. Again, most of this research is highly debatable. So, what's right for you?

I'm going to sit on the fence and hope I don't get splinters. I would say the choice - as always - is yours. If you find yourself in need - and can't stand the thought of black coffee, green tea, or water - grab yourself a flavored, sugar-free drink. **It's important that you stay normally hydrated**. I don't want you to make the mistake of the *Ramadan* researchers, and blame tiredness on fasting. **Be mindful that sugar-free drinks could still contain caffeine**.

What about chewing gum? There's no doubt that *chewing* itself starts up a *Pavlov's Dog* type reaction. Saliva will be produced in extra amounts, and **your stomach might anticipate a food arrival**. This in turn *could* promote a change in hormones. And, it's never good to trick hormones. My advice is - if you like gum - just chew it around meal times. By the way, brushing your teeth is fine at any time.

DRINKING FOR BOREDOM

In any of the plans - if you're successful at beating hunger - you might *still* need help with *boredom*.

The "B" word is not to be underestimated, even though it often is. Although it's not much, **drinking during your fasting periods might reduce boredom**. Hot drinks can be particularly welcome during cold times, or just at times when you need comfort in general.

There may be a *tiny* amount of calories in the drinks that you choose. We're talking 1 or 2 calories, or perhaps up to 10. That's cool. **Such a small amount of energy won't wake up the "security guards" who monitor everything inside you**. Insulin - *a hormone mainly produced when you eat carbs* - should stay low. And if that stays *low*, your growth hormone rises *high*, and you'll continue burning body fat.

DRINKING DURING MEALS

Liquids easily fill the stomach, and there is some evidence to suggest this could increase a general feeling of satisfaction. Specifically, liquids seem to do their best when they're consumed *with* a meal. If this works for you, do it.

Don't worry about "diluting stomach juices". When you're on a fast day of 600 calories, your body won't let a splash or two stop it from going about the extraction of nutrients.

DRINKING ALCOHOL

Okay, this needs to be said. **You should *not* drink alcohol on your fast days**. Even pure alcohol like *Vodka* interferes with the way Intermittent Fasting works. **Alcohol is 7 calories per gram (fat is 9) and all too easy to glug**. Before you get the butler to pour you another, be aware that some alcohol contains plant versions of *estrogen*. This encourages the laying down of fat in both sexes. It splendidly fattens madam's thighs and the master's stomach.

Alcohol has two problems that could particularly affect those using Intermittent Fasting. ***Physically*, alcohol disrupts blood sugar control**. It makes your muscles *less* efficient at dealing with food, especially over time. This is works directly against the benefits of *The IF Diet*.

Psychologically, **alcohol causes a subtle drop in motivation**. If your motivation drops below a certain threshold, it's quite likely that you won't be able to stick to your plan.

On non fasting days, the choice to have alcohol is yours. Undoubtedly, **you will lose fat and build health *faster* if you're alcohol-free**. My instinct is to let you use *your* instinct. **The entire focus of this book is to guide *you* to find happiness**. If you want a drink, have a drink. Just don't live on the stuff, or let it dominate what should be a random mix of foods during your feed days. Cheers!

IF YOU NEED A REMINDER

- stay normally hydrated when fasting, and drink when you're thirsty

- coffee, green tea, water and sugar-free drinks reduce boredom and increase fullness

- alcohol is best avoided when you're fasting

IF I JUST EXERCISE

Exercise helps you lose weight, right? Here's the real deal. **Exercise - *by itself* - is terrible at helping you improve the appearance of your body**. If taken to extremes - say marathon running 100 miles per week - it definitely "works". Less extreme measures - even visiting the gym 5 nights per week but *without* paying any attention to the food side - will *not* cause dramatic changes in shape.

Doing that increases fitness and strength, but that's not what many sign up for. The world is full of people using traditional exercise as a way of shifting the muffin top. And as you may have noticed, there are still *lots* of muffin tops pounding our streets! When these hard workers don't see the changes they deserve, they assume the terrible trio (slow metabolism, average genes, bad luck), and give up.

This is a shame - because done correctly - exercise is useful. So why does exercise not always live up to its shiny image?

Well, calories aren't the whole story, but they make a difference if you're relying on them alongside a typical diet. And when it comes to miles per gallon, the human body wins eco friendly awards year after year. It's an extremely efficient machine. Let me explain.

On average, jogging a mile uses about 100 calories. Sound good? Before you agree, consider that **a pound of your chub contains 3500 calories**. This means, **every pound of fat contains enough energy to jog 35 miles**. It doesn't seem like a fair deal to me, especially considering the sweat involved. And even if this mathematics appeals to you, it only works if nothing else changes in your life. As you'll see in a sec, that's quite unlikely.

PROBLEMS WITH TRADITIONAL EXERCISE

Exercise makes you hungry. If you slip into your *Nikes* and do some traditional exercise, you're highly likely to eat more calories than if you'd stayed in your regular shoes.

Researchers who disagree quote habits from a lab setting. **In the real world, traditional exercise - walking, jogging, swimming and weights - *cause* an overall increase in appetite**. And as *you* probably realize, **appetite can make or break your success**.

Appetite is deeply driven by the hormones we've had since day one. Cave living was a tough 200,000 year downturn, with food access being rare. So, your brain evolved a safety mechanism. If it sensed you'd been moving for a long time, steadily depleting your blood sugar - *and not replacing it* - something was wrong. Either food was in short supply, or you were a useless hunter. **This is what your brain senses during traditional exercise.**

The body responds by making you hungry, and tired. Tiredness stops you from wasting any more energy. Of course, **traditional exercise also causes us to overeat for a much simpler reason: we think we've earned it**. One definition of *junk food* is food you think you've *earned* from doing a bit of exercise.

This well-meaning binge is extremely common in today's health culture. Don't get sucked in.

Traditional exercise also takes up a lot of time. Visiting a gym - depending on its location - could steal a big chunk of your day. There are potential time issues with getting there and back, showering, and sometimes, waiting to use equipment. **Exercise programs that last for more than an hour often cause people to give up**. Year after year, gyms are packed out in January and Feb, then become ghost towns 'til early summer.

Even if you work out at home, traditional exercise isn't the smartest approach. Many people will be drawn to this book because it offers an *efficient* way to control body weight and improve general health. **Traditional exercise isn't efficient**. When you fast, you're already committing to improvement, and asking you to slog the equivalent of 50 laps around a track might tip your tolerance over the edge.

For guys, **traditional exercise can dramatically *reduce* hormone production**, including *testosterone*.

This is bad news, as testosterone affects everything from muscle to mood. For guys *and* girls, traditional exercise can also increase the chance of injuries, simply due to overuse (and the simultaneous lack of recovery). If you get injured, there's always a chance you'll mope around and overeat, or even avoid exercise from then on.

Now, don't get me wrong. For some people - especially those with a good and steady weight - exercise offers substantial benefits. We know what these are: **less disease**, **slightly longer life**, **higher self confidence**, **stronger immunity**, and a whole host of obvious and extensively researched benefits. Great. But for those reading this book, and for those intending to use it, traditional exercise just isn't the smartest place to start. So, what is?

Interval training is exercise that uses *short bursts* of effort, and spaces them out with *rest periods*. In many ways, it sounds like a cousin of Intermittent Fasting itself. And it's a good match too, a definite soul mate. Like the principles backing *The IF Diet*, interval training has been around for a long time, but only recently has it started to gain mainstream acceptance. The science behind it is solid, it works fast, and it's fun.

Originally designed to enhance the performance of athletes, **interval training will also *give* you heaps of energy, improve your health, and boost the effects of Intermittent Fasting itself**. And importantly, it will do this without taking up too much of your time. I won't pretend that it's easy. It's not. **It *is* the smartest, most efficient use of your sweat**. The results are impressive, and noticeable fast enough to keep you interested.

To use it, I recommend you get a general health check up first. Why? Because it's intense! Don't let that scare you, because once you get the go-ahead, **interval training is actually the *best* form of exercise to prevent serious health problems**. But obviously, if you have muscular or joint problems, or have a pre-existing heart condition, you need to get checked out first.

Compared to traditional exercise of a lower, slower intensity, interval training puts the body under real pressure. As a result, **the heart muscle itself grows stronger**. When you're not training, your new and improved heart will handle more regular demands *with ease*. **Arteries get worked hard, and they adapt by becoming more elastic**. More elastic arteries mean better head to toe blood flow - and possibly - a greater resistance to heart attacks.

Because you won't be training for long periods, **interval training doesn't stress out your hormone or immune system**. In fact, they get a *boost*. Only intense bursts of all-out effort cause a surge in growth hormone.

This hormone further increases fat burning, increases muscle tone, increases tendon strength (they join muscle to bone), increases ligament strength (they join bone to bone) - and - it firms your skin nicely.

Cellulite is affected by *how much body fat you have* - relative to what you were *designed to carry* - and *the quality of your skin*. Intermittent Fasting will help you get to a good weight, and interval training - through its growth hormone boosting power - will enhance your skin's collagen and elastin content. *Collagen & elastin* are the *bricks & cement* of your skin. The more you have, the less skin wrinkles and dimples.

Interval training - unlike traditional exercise - will *not* increase appetite dramatically. If you're doing it hard enough, you'll want to grab some water after, but that's about it. When you've finished a session of interval training - **the benefits will continue for hours** - even if by then you've forgotten about the training entirely. In fact, the increase in your metabolism and all its benefits mainly occur when you're *not training*.

When you work muscles intensely, there isn't time to get much fuel and oxygen into them. Keep pushing, and your body *must* use stored carbohydrate that's already *inside the muscle*. It's called **glycogen**. When you *burn* glycogen, your body will also "feel the burn" by producing **lactic acid**. This chemical tells us to *slow down*. There's only a small amount of glycogen inside saved up in each muscle, and your brain worries about it running out.

You'll never be able to run out of it completely (because it gets too painful), but the more you get rid of, the better. Burning up your glycogen tells your body that you mean business. **Food eaten in the hours after interval training will be directed to restocking muscles**. This makes it *much* less likely for *future food* to be converted into fat. Remember, food converted into fat can stay locked up for days, months, years, *or even a lifetime*.

Intense activity makes muscles ultra absorbent of carbohydrate. Think of interval training as squeezing water out of a sponge.

A dry sponge is more likely to soak up liquid, and that includes any excess carbs that float around your blood. Less intense training - *that's traditional exercise* - never matches these benefits. **Interval training closely resembles how we would have hunted as cave people**.

Because interval training turns your muscles into sensitive sponges, your body doesn't need to produce *as much* of the hormone insulin. Insulin's day job involves taking excess carbs out of the blood, and escorting them inside muscles. Insulin's *other* job, is taking excess carbs out of the blood, and converting them *into* fat itself. Can you see the bigger picture? **Make your muscles like sponges - reduce the need for insulin - reduce fat production**.

Now, once your muscles are brilliant at absorbing carbs, your body won't need to keep too much of them in the blood. Most people's muscles are so bad at absorbing carbs from the blood, that their body gets forced to keep levels high *all the time*. This causes the body to pump out *more* insulin. **Too much insulin will age anything, including organs**.

Eventually, the organ producing insulin takes early retirement, and you get *Type 2 Diabetes*.

Okay, I think I must have convinced you to give interval training a go. After you've done your first session and decided it's not worth it, read the whole chapter again! By the way, interval training is sometimes described as **HIIT**, which stands for *High Intensity Interval Training*. Same thing. Don't let the "High Intensity" words scare you either. Everyone starts somewhere. I will now cover the basics to get you started.

SADDLE UP

The most reliable way to get the benefits of interval training is to use a bike. That's where most of the research has been carried out. And by bike, I mean an *exercise* bike. You could use a *real* bike, but that would need perfect surroundings, including the complete absence of traffic (vehicles, humans and maybe horses). An exercise bike is something almost anyone can ride, and it allows you to focus on the most important thing: **effort**.

Total workout time **30 minutes**

Number of workouts **6 maximum**

- warm up is built in

- 3 minutes strolling followed by 4 minutes hard walking / repeated 4 times

- cool down for two minutes

At the risk of completely contradicting myself, this beginner program must *not* be done on a bike! It's best done by walking, either *outdoors* or using a *treadmill*. It will gently introduce your heart, lungs and muscular system to sudden changes in intensity. Even though I used the word *gently* earlier, it doesn't mean the actual exercise is. **If you do any interval training - *gently* - you'll reduce the benefits**.

This program isn't *true* interval training. But, it's what your body needs to get adjusted to.

If you find it too easy, skip it. The sooner you get to *the third program*, the better. Especially if you're following everything else in *The IF Diet*. **Perform this routine *whenever* you can. After 6 *workouts* - however long this takes - move onto the program after it**. The goal is to really get you motoring, and not spending too long working out.

TREADMILL METHOD

If you're going to use a treadmill, it will be simple to monitor how much is hard, and how much is easy (by looking at *speed*). **If you've never used a treadmill before, don't be scared**. They take a little getting used to, almost like learning to walk again. Fortunately, your brain and nervous system do this with just one workout. When you first get *off* a treadmill, it may feel slightly odd. That goes.

From the minute you first use one, **avoid holding on anywhere with your hands**. This massively limits the amount of muscle tissue used, because you stop using your chest, back, shoulder and arm tissue.

Holding on also reduces the use of muscles around your stomach and lower back, simply because they don't need to work. If none of this convinces you, just remember, you don't walk around in real life with your arms locked out like a mummy!

If it has the ability, **incline the treadmill (raise it up) by 1.5 degrees**. This *slight tilt* helps mimic the experience of walking outdoors. Apart from that, you don't need any fancy settings or automatic programs. Just hit the "Manual" or "Quick Start" button equivalent. **You will need to self-select an appropriate speed**. What's that? Difficult to say, because we're all different sizes, physical styles, and abilities.

In real terms, your *stroll* speed will probably be between **2.5 to 4 miles per hour** (4 to 6.4 kilometers per hour). I like the word *stroll* because it accurately describes the feeling you should have when doing it. For the *all out* fast part of the interval, I still want you *walking*, but quickly. The definition you should *feel* is "it almost feels like I'm running"! You want the feeling of being *close to taking off*.

"Close to taking off" is your ideal walking speed.

Apart from this, it's all quite simple. You start by *strolling* for 3 minutes. You then bump up the speed, and fine tune it until you're walking *hard*. You keep that going for 4 minutes. It may take a workout or two, but you'll soon get better at picking a speed that makes it difficult to *just last* the 4 minutes. There will be times that using the same speed as before feels harder *or* easier. Don't worry. **It's truly about *effort in the moment***.

When you finish blasting your way through a tough 4 minutes, you take the speed down to something that feels comfortable. It should *feel* like your legs are still moving, but not much more. I want you just to "keep the cogs turning". The real effort is in the fast 4 minutes. And again, please don't be tempted to hold on to the front or the sides of the treadmill. It actually can slow down recovery. Once you finish the - **3 minutes strolling & 4 minutes all out** - combination, you do it three more times, and cool down for a couple of minutes. *That's it.*

If you can push a little harder next time, great. Or, if work has tired you and lessens your speed, no worries. It's just about the relative *effort*. **After you've done this workout 6 times, you should move onto something more appropriate** (coming up after the *outdoor* version of this).

OUTDOOR METHOD

If you're venturing outdoors, you should have fun. If you're crossing streets, please be careful. A flat park could be ideal, but you will know what suits you best, based on enjoyment, safety, and practicality. The timings are identical to the treadmill version. All you need to know about is speed. Obviously, a stroll is just a stroll. There is no scientific way to describe it. Perhaps it's *just* faster than you walking along with a small child.

And for the fast part of the interval, walk *hard*. **What's "hard"? The speed you walk at *in a hurry*.** I don't want you to break into a jog or run. The purpose of these workouts is to get used to interval training *proper*, which comes soon.

If you've ever walked a dog that's been cooped up housebound for days, *that's* the speed you need! Will people stare at your sudden changes of speed? Maybe. They'll be staring at your good body soon.

INTERVALS FOR INTERMEDIATES

Total workout time **27 minutes**

Total number of workouts **12 maximum**

- **warm up for three minutes**

- **1 minute hard followed by 1 minute easy / repeated 10 times**

- **cool down for five minutes**

Once you've got those beginner intervals out of the way, you will be ready for a bit more *intensity*. As a human body gets fitter, it gets *more* able to demand *more* of itself. So, **while training does get easier, it also presents you with an opportunity to make it harder**. This workout is harder.

The hard parts are 1 minute long, and so are the easy parts. This is the perfect stepping stone towards the workout that follows this.

TREADMILL / OUTDOORS / ON THE SADDLE

You can do this workout on a *treadmill*, go *outdoors*, or use an *exercise bike*. Walking feels different to using the bike, but **all methods stress your body inside**. And yet again, it's about the *effort* you put in. The instructions should be fairly clear. Warm up for three minutes. Then, do one minute of *hard* peddling or walking, followed by one minute of *easy* peddling or walking. You repeat this sequence 10 times, and cool down for five.

Judging the intensity of the hard efforts can be difficult in the beginning. You might find yourself pushing hard in the early ones, and feel you're too exhausted to complete the last few. Or you could find yourself on the 10th effort, wondering if you could have pushed harder. After a few workouts, you'll get the hang of it.

With all interval training - be honest - and push yourself as hard as you can.

The relatively short 1 minute bursts will make your legs and calves *burn*. **This is lactic acid, produced because you're burning carbohydrate inside the muscle**. You will feel pain, and you will have loud breathing. This is normal. **If you ever feel chest tightness, stop immediately, and tell someone**. Done correctly, interval training is the thing that will *prevent* serious health problems from developing.

When you feel lactic acid burning in your lower body, you'll be producing growth hormone. The wonder juice will make your body slimmer *and* firmer. Lactic acid is also a very good indicator of how hard you *should* be pushing. **If you're pushing hard enough, you should be on the edge of lactic acid pain, and gritting your teeth to fight it**. This threshold is the *optimal* level to work at, *regardless* of the displayed treadmill or bike speed.

This level of training is quite a step up from the previous workout. Many of you won't be used to working so hard. Please, have faith. **After a short time, your body will start some incredible adaptions to help you out**. It will grow more blood vessels, more blood to fill them, more enzymes to break down fat at high speed, more enzymes to break down internal carbs at high speed, and, more muscle fibers to handle the effort. **You *will* get better**.

After you have completed 12 workouts of this kind, it's time to step it up. **Your body will be substantially improved inside** - and even if you don't see the outside changing quickly - it will catch up. As you continue to use *The IF Diet* - and interval training when you can - your entire system will work better as one perfectly co-ordinated unit. It does not take long to make this happen, assuming you work honestly, and with **effort**.

Total workout time **8 minutes**

Total number of workouts **Just keep going!**

- **warm up for two minutes**

- **hard 20 seconds followed by easy 10 seconds -
repeated 8 times**

- **cool down for two minutes**

In 1996, a Japanese researcher called *Izumi Tabata* discovered that super short periods of all-out effort - followed by short rests - could boost an athlete's fitness massively. In fact, they achieved levels of fitness that normally came from using a much longer time in the gym (*hours* in fact). The benefits of this training style were then explored by other researchers, keen to find general health benefits from such a short period.

I choose this method because even though it was designed to improve *fitness*, **Tabata training is brilliant for changing the physiology of the body *alongside* Intermittent Fasting**. Oh, and it's *fun*. Fun should never be forgotten when it comes to working out. It is a pleasure and privilege to have working arms and legs - so make use of 'em - and train like a smiling dog! *Tabata* training is physically and mentally challenging, but that in itself is *fun*.

ON YOUR BIKE

Tabata **training must be done on an exercise bike**. If you read up on the subject, you'll find lots of programs which use elliptical trainers (cross trainers), rowers, machine weights, dumbbells, kettle bells and climbers. **These are not suited to *Tabata* training**. They require too much co-ordination and don't allow you to focus on **all-out *effort***. Can't afford the gym? I would strongly consider getting an exercise bike. Save up. **It's an investment in your *life***.

The system is simple. Adjust the bike so you're comfortable. So you feel *strong*. Warm up for two minutes, *lightly*. You just want to get the hot blood moving around to loosen you up. Pause. Take a sip of water if you're nervous (you don't need it for hydration). Get ready, and **pedal like you're escaping from an angry dinosaur!** The bike may shift from side to side - *and you may look crazy* - but you'll be working correctly.

Judging how much effort to put in for the 20 seconds is hard, *if you plan it*. **So the simple thing is to be honest and go all-out**. In the first few workouts, your brain and body may hold you back. As you get fitter and more **effort confident**, you'll be able to push harder than before, and even surprise yourself with a smile! By the 8th interval, you should be *gasping* for air. Actually, that should start by about the 4th interval.

On the "easy" rest periods of 10 seconds - *relax* your peddling down (probably around **50 to 60 RPM** if the bike displays this) - but *continue* to move your legs.

This is important - as it *shifts blood* around - *removes waste*, and makes it *less of a shock* to start peddling hard again. To keep count of time, either look at the bike's display, use an egg timer, or get a *Tabata* phone app. Most of these apps are free, and sound an audible "beep" to guide your efforts.

You may think that *just* 8 minutes is a gimmick. I can assure you, it's the complete opposite. In fact, it's traditional exercise that's a gimmick in comparison. The main things to master are the principles of Intermittent Fasting itself. But if you are going to exercise - *and I suggest you give it a go* - interval training is undeniably the way forward. **Many people secretly dismiss it because it's hard**. Be smarter than them. Be honest.

WHY AND WHEN

Some of you might be wondering whether you should exercise *at all*. Certainly, if you follow *The IF Diet*, you will lose weight and improve your general health without exercise. If that's what you can manage, *that's what you can manage*.

I don't want you to start adding stuff if it makes you feel overloaded. As feelings based creatures, feelings are important. Maybe come back to exercise another time. Do come back though.

If you *have* got time, you might be wondering what kind of difference exercise *could* make. Honestly, I can't give you figures. If I did, I'd be guessing. But, **studies prove that people can lose weight with diet alone - although those who *add* exercise - tend to keep it off longer**. Is the exercise keeping the weight off, or do people exercise when they're already committed to keeping weigh off in the first place? Who knows.

From real life experience, **dietary change produces the biggest change**. There's no denying it. But **exercise undeniably increases feelings of self-esteem**. Exercise feels like a constructive force in life. It helps you feel like you're moving *forwards*. That moving forwards feeling is infectious, and it could well be something that helps you make positive decisions about *everything*. **If you have the time, save some for exercise**.

And speaking of time, that's another key question. How much time should you hand over to exercise? Well - as we've just seen - 8 minutes is enough time to really get things moving. **Interval training, particularly *Tabata* training, is physically tough on your muscles. I would suggest using it a maximum of *three* times per week, and *never more than two days in a row*.**

If you are going to give exercise a shot - and I'm referring to interval training - you might want to know what the *minimum* dose should be. **The minimum dose for interval training, is doing it when you can**. This is certain to annoy some sport scientists. Okay, in practical terms, by interval training *twice* per week, you will increase fitness and general health consistently, and measurably.

But - even if you do it *once* per week or *when you can* - it will help more than if you did *none at all*. I'm not trying to be smart. **Anything *is* more than nothing**. And in terms of it helping your diet-driven weight loss, it's possibly *much more*.

You see, if you exercise an average body, using an average diet, and use a below average frequency of exercise (once per week), you *will* get below average results.

***The IF Diet* quickly produces an above average body chemistry**, *before* your body even looks the part. If you exercise hard - even once per week - with *that* body, you will get above average results. Which brings me neatly on to the subject of *timing*. When to do your interval training. You may accuse me of trying to be smart again: **exercise when it best suits you**. This gives you the greatest chance of doing it again and again.

If you want to know the *ideal* time - physically speaking - here it is. **Intense exercise around the time that you're fasting will produce the greatest results**. Critics may immediately scoff at the idea of training when you're fasting. Remember, I'm not talking about *long duration exercise*. **I'm talking about 8 minutes**. Four hundred and eighty seconds. Okay, that does exclude transport or getting ready time. But seriously, 8 minutes.

If you exercise intensely - *around the times that you're fasting* - you'll produce *more lactic acid* and *more growth hormone*. You will reduce the amount of stored carbohydrate (glycogen) in your muscles *dramatically*. **Interval training enhances the effect of fasting periods**. Do them together, and you get **synergy**. Synergy is where you add one thing to another, and get more than you bargained for. A kind of **1 + 1 = 3** scenario.

Of course - when you *first* try fasting - you may feel too tired to exercise. As you progress with *The IF Diet*, fasting gets easier. And if you progress to the 8 minute *Tabata* training, you may find you have *more* mental energy. **Ideally, you'd exercise *before* food**. On *Thirder*, you'd slot it in an hour before your 8 hours of eating starts. On *Switcher* and *Weekender*, you'd do it an hour before the first *or* second of your meals.

Why do it an hour before? ***After* you finish blasting away, your body produces all kinds of enzymes and chemical enhancements which help it absorb future food quickly**.

If you *don't* eat for 60 minutes, these enzymes and chemicals continue to bubble up nicely (including growth hormone). **Do your interval training - wait about an hour - then eat**. That's enough. Longer waits could slow recovery, making your next workout *drag*.

So there you have it, **interval training, the perfect exercise complement to *The IF Diet***. It's not easy, but seeing the results will be. Start slowly, be honest with how hard you push, and keep getting better. Train when you can, up to three times per week. **If you can't manage it, come back to it another time**. Once you get comfortable with *Tabata* training, try it out at fasting times, an hour before you start eating.

SHOULD I DO WEIGHTS?

Weight training is a useful activity. The benefits are well documented. Building muscle improves shape, posture and bone. And, because muscle tissue burns calories, having *more* means having the potential to burn *more* calories **even while you're asleep**.

If you can hit the weights, *great*. It isn't an essential part of *The IF Diet*, and it needs a book of its own. You will lose lots of fat and noticeably improve your body *without* weight training.

If you *do* weight train - and do it when you use this book - here's some advice. On *Thirder*, train either *just before* you start eating, or *well within* the 8 hour eating gap. On *Switcher* and *Weekender*, weight train *on* your feeding days. **Weight training requires a different recovery process to banging out 8 minutes on an exercise bike**. If you're pumping iron properly - *you will damage muscle tissue* - and that requires you eat normally *soon after*.

SPECIAL NOTICE REGARDING WEIGHTS

If you happen to be someone who likes using weights but *won't* consider interval training, **listen up**. Pumping iron is great for building muscle, improving posture, boosting bone mass, balancing blood sugar control, and elevating hormones. But **there is a definite downside, if that's *all* you do**.

You may have never read about this before, but it's extremely important that you read the next paragraph.

Weight training can increase the stiffness of your arteries, the very pipes that keep you alive. Researchers have discovered both a short-term effect, and longer term evidence. After doing weights, some arteries go into a very slight "shock". For reasons not clear at the moment - *though possibly related to breath holding* - arteries can develop a reduced ability to contract and expand. This makes it tougher for your heart to work efficiently.

To stop this, you need to do something *after* you've hit the weights. Either consider using the interval training programs here (*including* the cool down), or go for a 10 minute walk. **Weight training *by itself* could cause a permanent increase in the stiffness of your arteries.** Really, all it takes is a few minutes cardio *after* weights to condition your arteries back into their normal, happy and elastic selves.

IF YOU NEED A REMINDER

- traditional exercise by itself isn't ideal for losing weight

- interval training is a powerful assistant to boost *The IF Diet* results

- training around fasting times produces the most positive effect

IF YOU HAVE NO EXCUSE

If you want to play basketball, it helps to be tall. If you want to be a championship jockey, it helps to be small. The genes for *maximum* height are decided for you. Shooting hoops for the *Knicks* or saddling up around *Kentucky* depends *mainly* on your parents. So, why did I highlight *maximum* and *mainly* just now? Well, **your genes play a big role in your life**. This quick chapter is about how **your life plays a big role in your genes**.

FLICK THE SWITCH

Epigenetics is a new word to describe something that's been happening for ever. *Charles Darwin* knew a lot about genes, but he didn't work this stuff out. The *Epi* part of *Epigenetics* is Greek, and it means "on top of". *On top of your genetics*. **Epigenetics is what happens when *nature* meets *nurture*.** And with our new understanding of genetics, we see that daily habits can make a bigger difference than DNA itself.

In the 1980s, a researcher wanted to see if good or bad harvests had made any difference to the health of children in a small Swedish county. Very accurate historical records made this possible. As it turned out, there were health differences depending on which era the children had grown up in. But there was a bigger surprise. **The variations in harvests had made noticeable health differences in those children's, children's children!**

Grandchildren of those who had lived during bad harvests, lived 6 to 32 years longer than those grandchildren who descended from times of good harvests. That wasn't a typo - **6 to 32 years difference** - depending on how the calculations were done. We now know that a pregnant mother's habits can affect her child's development for life, even though in theory, the child's genes would be fixed by that point.

This breakthrough sparked huge interest, and researchers looked to see if nurture could affect an individual during their *own* lifetime. They did this by studying those with matching genes.

Identical twins. Soon they discovered that in identical twins who had been separated *after* birth, genetic problems only "happened" in one of them. For example, asthma. Both twins had the gene, but only one got it.

It's like we're always playing catch-up with the subject of genes. First we discovered them. It wasn't enough. Then we mapped the entire human genome, the whole blueprint for building a human. It wasn't enough. Then we realized that even if you had certain genes, they might not be "expressed" in the real world. It wasn't enough. Actually, it is! **We now know that life deals us some cards, but how we play them is even more important**.

So - if you want to beat the banker - the first step is to realize that *you can*. Life deals you a complex set of genetic playing cards. Perhaps thousands of them. Each one is like a little switch, and **whether you have a healthy and happy life - or not - depends mainly on how smartly you play**. There are genes "for" obesity, and all the other factors connected to it.

But, we know that living correctly *can* overcome any bad cards you might have been dealt.

There are two changes of behavior that can strongly affect how your genes express themselves. **Intermittent Fasting will help you get to a correct weight, and being the correct weight itself may improve epigenetic factors**. In addition, **vigorous exercise will directly up regulate good genes, and suppress bad ones**. Interval training is without doubt the best way to induce these changes.

Early research on obesity found genes connected to blood sugar control, appetite, the "OB" gene, leptin levels, Brown Adipose Tissue (BAT), and various other complex sounding chunks of science. **We have now found that the environment - and that includes *us* - affects all of these**. Ideally, you'd be smart and pick better parents. Seeing the difficulty in that, I'd **stay optimistic by realizing how powerful your actions are**.

I have taken some cutting-edge science and dramatically simplified it for this section. My apologies to the geneticists reading this. But, I want the public to realize that while genes exist, their relevance in the world depends on how they interact with them. **Do not give your genes more power than they deserve - for 99.9% of humans, there are no excuses - it's *you* who has the final say**.

IF YOU WANT A REMINDER

- genes exist

- epigenetics exist too

- how you live could be more important than what you've been given

IF YOU KEEP GOING

Many people wonder if Intermittent Fasting is sustainable. It is. *Completely*. The more you do it - the slimmer and healthier you'll get - until you reach a natural limit. When you reach that point, you'll look and feel *fantastic*. **And you can stay there for as long as you want**. Your blood sugar control will be brilliant, and you would have gotten results *without* restricting food choices. You'll have no cravings, and you shouldn't feel like bingeing.

If for some other reason* you choose to stop, you'll *gradually* go back to normal. What's normal? Whatever you were before. Are you sighing with frustration? Don't. I guarantee you, **all other diets will return you to *worse* than normal and do it quickly**. They'll also leave you with a raging appetite, and a drop in mood. With Intermittent Fasting, the journey is so good - that if you hop off - you've got a chance to step back on with ease.

Its beautiful design is based on *our* beautiful human design. All other styles of living ("diets") move people away from that. If you move away from Intermittent Fasting, you're moving away from your own design. Remember the undeniable facts: fasting has been around since we have. **The IF Diet is not a "lifestyle choice" - *The IF Diet* is a "design choice"**. Big difference.

As research continues - and improves - we might find ways to enhance what we already know. But, it's unlikely that *any* discoveries will contradict our human design. In fact, that's a smart way to test *discoveries*. Whenever you're confronted with one, ask yourself the simple question, "Does this feel logical to me?". Your instinct - *that's the combination of all your knowledge filtered into a 1 second thought* - will guide you.

ONCE YOU ARE PERFECT

If you have hit your target - and look exactly as you want - you may be able to maintain *by doing less*.

It's a process of trial and error, **but many people find that by practicing the principles of Intermittent Fasting *one day per week*, they can keep all their success**. With respect to *The IF Diet*, I would say this advice definitely applies to the *Switcher* and *Weekender* plans.

If you're on *Thirder*, you'd need to maintain differently. It relies on a daily, temporary, and *moderate* restriction of feeding. This is different to the way *Switcher* and *Weekender* work. If you like the *Thirder* plan, you could try maintaining by using it for about 50% of your time. That would mean using it for 3 or 4 days out of every 7. By the way, there's nothing wrong with using the original plan on a continuous, lifetime basis.

I would also suggest that at least one day per week, you challenge yourself with some *vigorous* exercise, ideally interval training. **To help prevent sudden death and improve your general wellbeing, really favor the short, sharp shock of interval training**.

Get yourself checked out - and then *give your all* to peddling away on a bike - even if it's just **8 minutes per week**. You'll have another 10,072 minutes spare for other stuff. The bottom line is this. You can see *The IF Diet* as a way of shifting the fat. See it as, *a diet*. But beyond that, remember that Intermittent Fasting boosts *autophagy*, and that alone will help you look younger externally, and even internally. **By giving your body regular breaks from food - and that can even mean just *one* day per week - you'll help maintain your general health for *life*.**

IF YOU NEED A REMINDER

- *The IF Diet* is a system that fits your body's design

- you could maintain possibly on just 1 day per week

- if your focus is on weight don't forget about health

* Sometimes life throws us a curveball. With 7 billion humans roaming the planet, there's bound to be a complicated situation at one time. If such a time arrives, there's a good chance that keeping slim and healthy will lose its charm. More worrying stuff will occupy your thoughts. **Don't beat yourself for this**. It's called *life*. Just deal with your priorities as best you can, and get back to it when you're free of anxiety. The science will still be there, waiting for you with open arms.

IF ANYONE ASKS

If friends, family or co-workers ask what you're doing, don't be afraid. I know, you might get some strange looks. You may even get discouragement. To be fair, it's understandable.

Intermittent Fasting marches against our much hugged modern ideas of what's healthy and sensible.

If only everyone realized that this smart 21st century is a mere blink of an eye compared to how long we've roamed the planet. If you're on *Thirder*, and have chosen to shift your 8 hour eating gap to suit your evenings, you might be skipping breakfast. I know and *you* know that you will *break* your *fast*, just a bit later. **Others might worry for you**, assuming chaos will come from not having your morning *Cheerios* medicine. And if you're on *Switcher* or *Weekender*, random friends might pop by and wonder why you're not "eating normally".

The point of *The IF Diet* is to do what other diet books don't do, and that includes every other book on Intermittent Fasting.

It's point is to give you a choice, a way of doing something clever for your body, *without* it affecting your enjoyment of life. And that includes, *not* upsetting your friends and family. No man is an island. We *need* others. **Find a way of making this work**, and respect the curiosity that others have about this.

IF YOU NEED A REMINDER

- be prepared to be questioned about *The IF Diet*

- respect others' curiosity and get them to read up

- if you simply become fabulous the criticism will stop!

IF YOU WANT TO GIVE UP

Do it. You weren't expecting that! *The IF Diet* isn't about rules. You make those. And, it's definitely not about me giving you pep talks or spouting psychobabble. **If you find yourself wanting to give up, it means you've lost your motivation**. And if you've lost that, there's no point in you just fighting against it. A loss of motivation happens for a reason. **You just need to find out what it is - regroup - and go again when *you* are ready**.

WE'RE EXPERIENCING TECHNICAL ISSUES

The number one reason to lose motivation - especially on a diet - is things not turning out like you expected. If that's the case, feeling like giving up makes complete sense. But before you do that, **be utterly honest**. Are you doing everything correctly? Are those 600 calorie days actually 1200? Is your *Thirder* 8 hour feeding gap occasionally 14? If you re-read the chapter on genetics, you'll be reminded that we can't blame much on them either.

Before you think it, I haven't become a drill sergeant. I just don't want you giving up for weak reasons. Diets - and that's all diets - aren't out to get you. They are basic structures of **cause and effect**. Do *this* and you'll get *that*. If something isn't working, it probably just needs *slight* adjustment. Try writing your habits down for a week and looking at them after. It's not to show anyone else. I want *you* to look at *you*.

MY PYRAMID IS BROKEN

2013 marks the 70th anniversary of a little research paper called *A Theory of Human Motivation*. In it, American psychologist *Abraham Maslow* published the results of his findings into **what makes humans tick**. He studied hundreds of people, focusing on those who had achieved excellence, including a certain *Albert Einstein*. Despite a mix of backgrounds, he kept finding common patterns of behavior.

He arranged these into an order, or what scientists call a *hierarchy*. Other psychologists adapted *Maslow's* findings, and arranged them into a pyramid.

That's why it's also called *Maslow's Pyramid*. His theory was simple. We need to fulfill our most basic needs (at the bottom of the pyramid), before we fulfill the needs at each level above it. If we didn't - we'd feel anxious - and never make much progress in life.

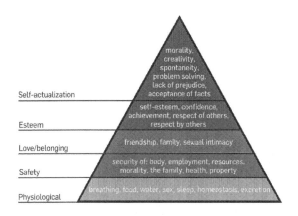

The theory makes a lot of sense. *Maslow* regarded the first 4 levels of the pyramid as "D needs", with the "D" standing for *deficiency*. If you didn't get them, you would be deficient, and you wouldn't achieve what was above it. From very basic physical functions at the bottom, it moved all the way up to *self actualization* (a rather posh way of saying *achieving one's potential*).

When it comes to dieting, I think his theory needs to be flipped upside down, literally.

You see, we live in a very different world to *Abraham Maslow*. We live in the age of *wanting more*, caused largely by being *hyper aware*. Newspapers, television, cinema and now the internet, make us compare ourselves to apes from every forest on the planet. This highly *un*-natural situation makes most modern humans develop **status anxiety**.

This means that we tend to worry about those things higher in the pyramid *earlier* than we should. If our life isn't on track, if our job is stressing us out, or if we're simply struggling to pay the bills, we get incredibly anxious. *Those* things cause us a loss of motivation, and *that* filters down into our more basic needs, especially *food* and *homeostasis*. Put simply, **we lose motivation to diet, because something else is up**.

If something is "broken" in your pyramid - you need to find out what it is - and deal with it. Once you've done that, you'll wipe out a huge chunk of anxiety, and be able to focus on your health again. This is why I don't believe in pep talks. There are no lazy humans, only unmotivated ones.

And a strong *lack* of motivation comes from having certain human needs *not* being met in key areas. Be honest, face them, fix 'em. Job done.

IF YOU NEED A REMINDER

- if you feel like giving up, take a break to review the situation

- if the diet isn't working for technical reasons, re-plan and go again

- if there are deeper problems in your life, fix these *first* and return to the diet after

IF YOU NEED A SUMMARY

Are we nearly there yet? We are! You have the lion's share of information, and all you need to do now is, **apply it**. It may have felt like you've been back to school with all the science, but it *is* important. If you start to doubt your sanity - or if others make you doubt it - just think back to the techy stuff. This is a real opportunity to improve your health. Here's a quick reminder of where you've been.

IF YOU WANT BACKGROUND STUFF

- diets can work for you if they're correctly constructed

- constantly cutting back on calories causes problems

- problems include muscle loss, boredom and weight regain

- intermittent fasting cuts calories in tune with our design

- this boosts fat loss, saves muscle, and improves health

- you can pick your own foods and don't have to exercise

IF YOU WANT PRACTICAL STUFF

- *The IF Diet* has 3 programs to choose from

- *Thirder* is eat normally but within an 8 hour gap

- *Switcher* is eat normally one day and eat 600 cals the next

- *Weekender* is eat normally on 5 days and eat 600 cals for the other 2

- at fasting times your 600 cals can be divided into 2 meals (3 in first week)

- you can drink coffee, green tea, water or sugar-free drinks at any time

IF YOU WANT EXTRA STUFF

- interval training even 8 minutes per week can boost results

- higher protein intakes with meals help control appetite

- food variety protects against disease and could boost fat loss

- genes make a difference but hard work is even more powerful

- you could maintain *The IF Diet* results with 1 day a week fasting

- if you find yourself struggling, be honest and push on regardless

1. Pick a plan!

2. Apply it!

3. Book a holiday!

IF I WANT MORE

Most of you will get great results from following the plans alone. And yet some of you will still want *more*. That's a great attitude, so keep it up. *The IF Diet* puts its chapters - and your priorities - in order. That's why this stuff is back here. **Experts may think this information is "basic"**. They're wrong. The basics are having the correct diet *design*. After all, the word *diet* is from the Latin for "way of life". **Always, always, always, get that right *first***.

If you're on *Thirder*, you may want to start looking at this section earlier than those on *Switcher* or *Weekender*. And if you're already on one of those - *once you have the fast days nicely integrated into your schedule* - take a look at these. They're a starting point, rather than absolute advice. When you feel like you can handle more, and really want to tighten up your non-fasting times, see if you can make these extra factors work for you.

Fiber is the rough stuff in food that we can't digest. There are two types, **soluble** and **insoluble**. Their definitions relate to whether they can be absorbed in water or not. **Both have benefits, and it's smart to seek a mix of fibers**. Fiber helps weight loss mainly through encouraging you to eat less calories in total. It especially does this on diets where there isn't strict control of calories. That's like Intermittent Fasting on non-fasting days.

High fiber foods *mechanically* help control your appetite. Soluble fiber particularly causes a mess within your stomach, which helps slow digestion from there onwards. Your blood sugar will rise slowly, which means a sudden *peak and crash* is less likely. Insoluble fiber also increases fullness.

Instead of naming specific foods, just remember if you see a *high fiber* option of your favorite food, check it out.

We briefly touched upon protein earlier in the book. Protein helps dieters, without doubt. The only doubt is *why*. **We know that protein appears to increase satiety**, a feeling of fullness and contentedness. And that's compared to carbs or fat. The mechanism is not currently clear. Protein could possibly be fulfilling an evolutionary role in our diet. Over half of your dry weight is protein, and it needs to be replaced on a daily basis.

If you eat too little protein, it could be harder to maintain your muscle mass.

And muscle mass is important, as it's the largest "user" of food. Protein is also **thermogenic**, which means it increase *heat production*. If you produce more heat - and lose it - you're losing energy. Burning calories! Again, protein does this better than carbs or fat. At non fasting times - forget studying labels - but **try to include some protein with your meals**.

We used to think that all sugars were created equal. They're not. Like many things in life, some stuff falls apart quickly, and some stuff stays strong. Carbohydrates are just the same. Their structure determines how easily absorbed they are in the human body. **Certain carbs get broken down very quickly, and therefore raise your blood sugar quickly**. The trouble comes when you do this too often.

Too much blood sugar makes the body panic. Why? Too much sugar in the blood can damage organs. To respond to this threat, the body churns out *insulin*. Insulin picks up the sugar, and takes it over to muscle *or* fat cells. Ideally - it takes more of it to muscle - where it can be used later. Unfortunately, **if you raise your blood sugar *too high* and *too often*, it's inevitable that your insulin will shovel it into fat cells, and make you chunky**.

Diabetics can have serious problems with their blood sugar control, so a scientist developed **a scale which measures the speed at which carbs raise blood sugar**. If you want, you can imagine it as a ranking of cars and their acceleration. He called this the **glycemic index**. Ranking pure glucose with a score of 100, everything else gets judged *relative* to that, in terms of how much a sugar rush it delivers.

Studies suggest that if you consistently eat *lower glycemic* food, you're more likely to be slim. Low glycemic foods keep your blood sugar stable, which in turn keeps insulin stable. And when insulin is stable, you tend to *use* your blood sugar, instead of converting it to fat. **Vegetables are almost always the lowest foods in a glycemic index**, as are protein rich foods like meat (because they contain few carbs, and it's carbs which most affect insulin).

Many years after developing the glycemic index, it began to be criticized by some scientists. They argued that the data was based on eating foods in isolation, and in a fixed amount.

Real life tends to mix all kinds of foods together, and in different portion sizes to those tested in labs. So, we invented a concept called **glycemic load**. In all honesty, it's too complex, and completely impractical. So, I mention it here just to acknowledge it.

I do recommend glancing at the glycemic index at least *once* in your life. Get a rough idea of how foods raise your blood sugar. The speed at which foods accelerate into your system is only one factor, but it can throw up surprises. Very few people would know that *French Baguette* bread raises blood sugar *faster* than table sugar. And of course, you rarely eat baguette by the teaspoonful! As I said, check it out (*Google* it) just once.

FRUCTOSE

Fructose is an interesting chap. It's even more curious, especially considering we've just chatted about the glycemic index. Fructose is very low on that, but acts very naughtily in the body.

Commonly known as "fruit sugar", it makes up a high percentage of the modern Western diet. It's naughty because it interferes with your insulin, and even your appetite. There's no point in obsessing over the stuff, but it's smart to be aware of its dangers.

When you eat fructose, it gets digested in the small intestine, and processed again by your liver. This form of absorption is different to many other sugars. Some research suggests that fructose makes insulin do a bad job. That's to say, **too much fructose reduces how muscles respond to insulin**. If muscles and insulin don't get on well, blood sugar keeps building up. And when *that* happens, you produce even more insulin.

Constantly raising insulin is not a good idea. Apart from making you fat, insulin *itself* could be linked to ageing your insides and your outsides. The latest research seems to find fructose guilty in another way. **Fructose confuses your appetite**. And when I say confuse, I mean, it lets it off the leash. Obviously if you're eating lots of calories in general, fructose's potential for appetite chaos, *goes up*.

Normally, as we eat food, we increase something called **leptin**. This hormone, from the Greek word for "thin", eventually tells your body to *stop eating*. **Fructose *stops leptin***. I'll say it clearly: **fructose stops your body from knowing when to stop eating**. At the same time, fructose can interfere with **ghrelin**. Ghrelin's job is to encourage us to eat. Once you eat something, it's supposed to go down. As I said, *supposed to*.

If you've ever eaten a meal *and still felt hungry*, this could be a problem due to fructose. Ghrelin drives us to eat - and once we've obeyed, we're supposed to feel content - and stop. Fructose somehow jams the Ghrelin signal, allowing it to stay high. With ghrelin high, your body still thinks it hasn't been fed. Couple that with turning off leptin (your body's fuel gauge), and you really just keep eating all the time.

Like everything in this section, it's just to make you aware. *The IF Diet* will go to war against your fat, but you can make the battle easier if you like. Fructose *does* occur naturally in fruits, but it's not a problem unless you eat (or drink) fruit all day long.

Besides, fruit comes packaged with vitamins, minerals, and good things we don't even have names for yet. If you want to cut down on something, **cut down on soft drinks**.

These used to be made with regular sugar, which ironically did less damage and tasted better. But fructose is *much* cheaper. In carbonated drinks, it's labeled **high fructose corn syrup** or **HFCS**. I don't blame the companies. If you were running *Coca Cola* - and selling **1 billion (1,000,000,000) cans of *Coke* a day** - wouldn't you pick the most economical ingredients? There's nothing like a crisp and cold *Coke* during a hot summer. Just don't live on it.

MEAL FREQUENCY

A few moments ago, we met **leptin**. When you eat meals, leptin rises in proportion, and tells your brain *to tell you*, "we're done here". Stop eating. We now know that **meals boost leptin better than snacks**.

In recent times, there has been a trend towards eating smaller, more frequent servings of food. Scientists and trainers argued this would lead to more stable blood sugar control, especially in comparison to eating larger meals less often.

Small meals - or snacks - do raise blood sugar less than bigger meals. That's obvious. But it's not *everything*. The *frequent meal theory* became popular at a time when *all we could do* was study blood sugar. We've done that for 100 years plus. **We discovered leptin in 1994!** And today's scientists *can* measure it, even though it's so small you wouldn't see it on top of a pin. **It seems that little leptin has more to say than blood sugar**.

If you're following *The IF Diet*, it's something to be aware of on non-fasting days. **Don't feel compelled to eat small frequent meals**. Many of us have been forced to eat against our instincts. Some of this was a genuine mistake, and at other times, it's been a way of selling us more snack food, and food in general. **You should easily be able to handle more than 3 or 4 hours between meals.**

If you can't, keep doing *The IF Diet* until you can!

Meals raise leptin correctly. Less frequent feeds result in longer gaps *between* meals, which is something that you keep hearing me mention. **Gaps between food allow your body to tap into its own energy source, body fat**. Finally, meals - *not snacks* - are social. Studies show that you eat *more* when you watch television, and *less* when you sit with good company. If you love eating while watching - balance it out - and sit *with* someone!

VITAMIN D

Vitamin D isn't actually a vitamin. Something is a vitamin if the organism can't produce it and needs to get it from diet. Vitamin D can be produced in our skin, assuming there are enough rays breaking through. So if you're going down the natural production route, it's best to be as naked as possible during spring and summer. And it helps to be less furry! **Approximately 20 to 30 minutes of light on skin produces good Vitamin D**. And?

In the body, Vitamin D affects hundreds of things. You might know it as something that boosts bone mass. It does. But it also helps your muscles become better at absorbing things from the blood. In particular, its relationship with the storage hormone *insulin* gets much better. This is called **improving insulin sensitivity**. Exercise does that, as does Intermittent Fasting. When your insulin works as it's intended to, fat loss improves dramatically.

Other than carefully enjoying the bright weather on your skin, I'd consider adding a bit more supplemental Vitamin D. Normally, I advise *against* targeting just one vitamin or mineral, because it's easy to unbalance other nutrients by doing that. **A sensible approach would be to take a quality multi-vitamin that contains at least 100% of the recommended daily intake for D**. If you take fish oils, they often contain some too.

FISH OILS

Some fat is very important. There are two fats - *Omega 3 & 6* - often called *essential*, because they are.

Having enough of these during and after pregnancy, and possibly even before pregnancy, helps guarantee a healthy child. **These essential fats are part of your eye and brain structures, and every cell wall throughout your body**. Science has found that a lack of Omega 3 & 6 in the diet could reduce your potential for burning fat.

When you increase these essential fats - especially Omega 3 - your cell walls tend to become more "fluid". They get better at *letting bad stuff out*, and better at *letting good stuff in*. This helps your muscles improve how they work with insulin. Yet again, improving the insulin and muscle relationship leads to many benefits. **You'll have more stable blood sugar, which means you should be better at controlling appetite**.

Indeed, appetite is also improved through Omega fats, because they seem to play a role in *depression*. **Being depressed often leads to emotional overeating. Our brains have a high percentage of Omega 3 fat, particularly one called Docosahexaenoic Acid, or DHA**.

When we examine the brains of depressed people, they tend to be quite low in DHA. **Correcting this deficiency over time could lead to a reduction in depression**.

Essential fats are found in the diet, particularly in cold water fish (*salmon, mackerel, trout*). You can also get small amounts in **walnuts**, and **flax seed oil** (sometimes called "linseed oil"). Supplements exist too, including vegetarian versions made from the **marine plankton** that floats on the top of oceans. In fact, **fish don't naturally contain any omega 3 *until* they eat plankton *which does***.

The benefits of Omega 3 fats are considerable, possibly because they formed a critical step in our evolution. At one point, cavemen would have eaten the brains of other species, and even the brains of other cavemen. This rapid re-concentration of Omega 3 fats definitely assisted in our mental development. Fortunately, you can now buy smashingly good pills of the stuff, rather than smashing your fellow Earth dwellers with a club.

If you asked, "what pill would you take if you could just take one?", I'd answer "**an Omega 3 supplement**". If I ate fish, I'd pick a multivitamin instead (I'm an animal loving vegetarian - including fish!). **If you *do* eat fish, 1 - 2 servings per week will do**. If you're a girl, you could get by on **15 to 30 ml of flax oil daily**. Men *don't* absorb flax well. Other than this, buy a decent fish / marine oil supplement. **Get one with 200mg - 600mg of DHA per day**.

FOOD

I thought I'd save the best for last. Do you like the glamorous subtitle? I know that being slim *isn't* just about eating less and exercising more. In fact, I hope this section underlines that. First, get the *design* of your diet right. That's using a plan from the book. And then - *if you can* - find ways to improve on the finer details. If you held a gun to my head and screamed "GIVE ME THE SECRET!", I'd calmly look you in the eye and say, "Food".

And when I say *food*, I mean the stuff closest to nature. The stuff that's been around since we have. A mix of modern factors including wars, famines and just plain old money making have made us brilliant at *making* food. Well, what we've actually made sometimes doesn't deserve the "F" word. Maybe if "F" stands for *Frankenstein*. **Real "food" is the stuff that your grandmother would have called "food"**.

If you want to know what true "food" is - ask this - "Will this thing in front of me stay fresh for more than a few days?". If the answer is "Yes", *it's not food*. Vegetables, fruits, and quality meats won't stay fresh for that long. Their nutrients are real, and they're fading the longer you leave them. And that, is a great sign. It's what *Mother Nature* intended. She wanted us to eat **locally grown (fresh)**, **chemical free**, *food*.

We're discovering more and more things in "food". Deficiencies in one *tiny* nutrient can cause *major* health problems. We often try and isolate these nutrients in our labs. We don't need to. **The grocery store is *your* laboratory**.

The most famous doctor in history - and perhaps the only one who understood the true value of food - was *Hippocrates*. Old Hippo had a great philosophy.

"Let food be thy medicine, and medicine be thy food."

When you're faced with a food choice dilemma, **just think food**. You are what you eat - and if you eat close to nature - you will be closest to nature's intended design. Of course, chocolate chip cookies are *highly* unnatural - and of course - they taste *highly* pleasurable! **Definitely, enjoy some of our delicious man-made treats**. That's just good life balance. But always remember where you came from, and consume a bit of that history, *every day*.

IF YOU NEED A REMINDER

- other factors can increase the effectiveness of any diet

- without *The IF Diet* in place these become more important

- be aware of the science and use it once you've mastered the basics

IF I WANT IT FAST

There will be times when you're out and about, and you need something to eat, *fast*. I've compiled a small list of foodstuffs from 6 of the major fast food restaurants, with each item being 300 calories or lower. **This list isn't meant to be advice on what to eat!** It's simply to make you **aware** of what's out there. And it's to let you know, that there *is* opportunity to have *fun on the run*. Remember, **food eaten on fast days will be processed very efficiently**.

Due to consumer pressure, most of the major food chains now *visibly* list calories on their in-store menus. And if you can't find the details in-store, the company website will certainly have what you need. **In fact, estimating the calorie content of food is now easiest *outside* the home**. Always eat a nice mix of foods if possible. After this section, you'll get the full extent of my advice regarding those magic 600 cals.

IF YOU WANT MCDONALD'S

Cheeseburger **295**

Two hash browns **280**

Hamburger **250**

Six pieces of Chicken McNuggets **250**

Small French fries **230**

Fish Fingers **195**

Oatso Simple Porridge **195**

Grilled chicken and bacon salad **190**

Garden side salad **20**

Regular tea with one milk carton **10**

Regular Diet Coke **4**

Regular black coffee **0**

IF YOU WANT KFC

BBQ wrap **300**

Zinger salad **290**

Mini fillet burger **289**

Regular Popcorn Chicken **283**

Two mini breast fillets **263**

Original Recipe salad **263**

Regular fries **247**

One piece Original Recipe chicken **244**

Three Hot Wings **243**

Large BBQ Beans **176**

Corn Cobette **150**

Pepsi Max 600ml bottle **2**

IF YOU WANT SUBWAY

Egg and Cheese Breakfast Sub **294**

6" Chicken and Bacon Ranch Melt **292**

Bacon Breakfast Sub **279**

6" Subway Melt **249**

6" Veggie Patty **247**

Pepperoni Pizza Toastie **247**

6" Steak and Cheese **245**

6" Tuna **233**

Country Chicken and Vegetable Soup **168**

Chicken Breast Salad **139**

Garden Side Salad **21**

IF YOU WANT DOMINO'S

Large Classic Crust slice of Americano **268**

Large Classic Crust slice of Full House **268**

Large Classic Crust slice of Veg-A-Roma **240**

Large Classic Crust slice of Pepperoni Passion **228**

Chicken Wings **227**

Chicken Strippers **224**

Large Classic Crust slice of American Hot **218**

Large Classic Crust slice of Domino's Deluxe **209**

Large Classic Crust slice of Hawaiian **203**

Large Classic Crust slice of Vegetarian Supreme **192**

Large Classic Crust slice of Cheese and Tomato **183**

Potato Wedges **149**

IF YOU WANT PIZZA HUT

Six pieces of Baked Hot Wings **300**

Four pieces of Traditional Lemon Pepper Wings **300**

Medium Pan Supreme slice **290**

Medium Pan Pepperoni Lover's slice **290**

Four pieces of Traditional Honey BBQ Wings **280**

Medium Pan Spicy Sicilian slice **270**

Medium Pan Pepperoni slice **250**

Medium Pan Cheese slice **240**

Medium Pan Ham and Pineapple slice **230**

Medium Pan Veggie Lover's **230**

Fit 'n' Delicious Chicken, Red Onion, Green Pepper slice **180**

Fit 'n' Delicious Diced Red Tomato, Mushroom and Jalapeno slice **150**

IF YOU WANT BURGER KING

Egg and Cheese Butty with Heinz Ketchup **300**

Sweet Chilli Chicken Wrap **296**

Regular Fries **291**

Hamburger **284**

BK Veggie Bean Burger **278**

Regular Mini Pancakes with Maple Syrup **269**

SIx Regular Chicken Nuggets **258**

Four Regular Chilli Cheese Bites **252**

BK Bacon Butty with HP Sauce **214**

BK Bacon Butty with Heinz Ketchup **213**

Flame Grilled Chicken Salad **128**

Garden Salad **33**

IF YOU NEED A REMINDER

- if you are fasting, fast food can still be healthy

- your body processes food efficiently when fasting

- always eat a variety of foods to maximize general
health

IF YOU KNOW BEST

Traditional diet books are packed with food suggestions. The "everything's included" style definitely helps them sell. Listen up. **It definitely won't help *you***. Being shown lists and asked to pick something does feel nice to begin with. It gives us a chance to assert our personality. But eventually - personalities need more space - and **we do what we like**. Now to me - that's a great place *to start* - especially if you're on *Switcher* or *Weekender*. Ready?

Eat - what - you - want. The science behind Intermittent Fasting is handing that to you on a plate, *literally*. **Dieters, rejoice in the FREEDOM that is 600 calories!** *The IF Diet* is all about freedom. Intermittent Fasting is all about freedom. Your chance of long-term success is *all about freedom*. **And the simplicity of choosing *your* 600 calories is all part of the fun**. Yes, I did just say "fun"! I think you need a clearer paragraph of *how-to* advice. Pay close attention.

On fasting days - eat up to 600 calories - you choose what. On fasting days - eat up to 600 calories - you choose what. On fasting days - eat up to 600 calories - you choose what. On fasting days - eat up to 600 calories - you choose what. On fasting days - eat up to 600 calories - you choose what. On fasting days - eat up to 600 calories - you choose what. On fasting days - eat up to 600 calories - you choose what.

Anyone who tells you *what* to eat on a day when you're hardly eating *at all* is missing the point. And I do regard a list of suggested foods and recipes as *telling you what to eat*. **There must be no limitations on the *600 calories* advice**. None. The minute your relationship to food is restricted beyond *one* piece of advice, everything starts to go wrong. **Find the 600 calories you enjoy. Nothing else matters**.

Pretty much every food today comes with a label. If you love food without labels, and don't know what's in something, the content is just a *Google* away. **Discovering is fun**.

Seriously, your right to choose does not need to be dumbed down any more. **My only rule is that you don't get 600 calories from alcohol**. Alcohol is just the name we give to different flavors of the chemical *ethanol*. On fast days, it's a no-no. Apart from that, **you choose**.

If you do get bored and *want* a recipe or suggestion for something around "X" calories, there are thousands at your fingertips. The internet isn't perfect, but it's much less restricted than some awful writer's taste bud preferences. I feel strongly about this because I've repeatedly witnessed the damage done *the minute food choice gets limited*. **Intermittent Fasting has the science to put the power in *your* hands, and that's where it needs to stay**.

Once you get a feel for calories and portion sizes, you will become an expert in your own right. And once you're an expert, you'll have the confidence of one. And once you've got confidence, you'll never have a reason to lose hope. One more "and". And once you have hope, you'll have anything you want.

A better body, a better mind, even a better life in general. **Believe in the power of *do-it-yourself*.** I do.

IF YOU NEED A REMINDER

- you don't need me to suggest your 600 calories

- on fasting days - eat up to 600 calories - you choose

- you will soon become an expert, full of confidence, and full of hope

IF YOU NEED HELP

If you get stuck or need motivation, there are many places to go. In 2013, most of us will start with our laptops, or phones. And there's nothing wrong with that, especially with such a fast developing science. But, I urge you not to stray too far from the programs in this book. There are some seriously whacky varieties around - and while they sound good - they're often based on *one* person's findings. Even non scientists know that's a risky strategy.

Having said that, **practical support is what most of us need**. Scientists rarely consider this, because most of their work is carried out in controlled conditions. Our world can be a wild one, and some of the best people to make sense of the chaos, *are* people. **Your fellow humans can be the best source of day-to-day advice**. They are the front line soldiers who really know *how stuff works*. If you're not sure, just ask someone.

As a front line soldier yourself, you have a very real part to play in winning the battle of the bulge.

Your success will be infectious, and it could *transform* a stranger's life. Spread the smiles and excitement by sharing your most useful tips, taking before and after photos (showing them too), and being supportive when you know you can. Helping out and co-operation is the stuff that makes being a human so special. Good luck!

Meet your like-minded & lovely fellow humans at:

facebook.com/ifdiet

IF YOU CAN PROVE IT

Technically, "proof" never exists. The best we have is *what most scientists agree with right now*. And to see what most scientists are agreeing on, you've got to hunt them down (they're way too busy to socialize). You do this by looking at research. It may initially look like a complicated mess of vaguely English words. With a bit of patience, I can assure you it's possible to learn the language known as *Modern Geek!*

The best research for humans, is research using humans. Annoyingly, the majority of research is still non-human. This is less than ideal, especially for the animals who are forced to help us discover things they have no interest in. Rather than exclude animal research, some is included. Ignoring their contribution would mean their efforts were wasted. In the meantime, **I urge you to push for commercial products that are free of animal testing**.

Finding research is relatively simple. A good starting point is the US government's free online database.

You can find the *National Institutes of Health* website at - **pubmed.gov** - and tap the 8 digit **PubMed ID** into the search box. Or just *Google* the study's official title. Under each one, I've put *my* plain English translation. Don't be scared of this stuff. **And never forget: the ultimate proof is for you to become *living proof*.** Go for it.

Alternate day fasting (ADF) with a high-fat diet produces similar weight loss and cardio-protection as ADF with a low-fat diet.

How IF feed days work well regardless of whether you use a high or low fat diet.

Metabolism: Clinical & Experimental in 2013

PubMed ID 22889512

Intermittent fasting combined with calorie restriction is effective for weight loss and cardio-protection in obese women.

How mixing IF and CR using liquid meals causes weight loss and boosts heart health.

Nutrition Journal in 2012

PubMed ID 23171320

The effects of intermittent or continuous energy restriction on weight loss and metabolic disease risk markers: a randomized trial in young overweight women.

How a 25% of normal calorie intake on alternate days creates effective weight loss.

International Journal of Obesity in 2011

PubMed ID 20921964

Improvements in coronary heart disease risk indicators by alternate-day fasting involve adipose tissue modulations.

How alternate day fasting reduces body fat, heart disease risk, and maintained muscle.

Obesity in 2010

PubMed ID 20300080

Short-term modified alternate-day fasting: a novel dietary strategy for weight loss and cardio protection in obese adults.

How eating 25% of calories on alternate days caused a weekly fat loss of 1.5 pounds.

American Journal of Clinical Nutrition in 2009

PubMed ID 19793855

Dietary and physical activity adaptations to alternate day modified fasting: implications for optimal weight loss.

How hunger and physical activity rapidly adapt by using IF and help weight loss.

Nutrition Journal in 2010

PubMed ID 20815899

Improvements in body fat distribution and circulating adiponectin by alternate-day fasting versus calorie restriction.

How IF produces the same benefits of CR in terms of body fat cell distribution.

The Journal of Nutritional Biochemistry in 2010

PubMed ID 19195863

Is periodic fasting really good for reducing cardiovascular risk and improving heart health?

How the mainstream medical establishment are reluctantly coming to terms with IF.

Future Cardiology in 2011

PubMed ID 22050055

Alternate-day fasting in non obese subjects: effects on body weight, body composition, and energy metabolism.

How fasting midnight to midnight on alternate days causes fat loss in non fat people.

American Journal of Clinical Nutrition in 2005

PubMed ID 15640462

Alternate-day fasting reduces global cell proliferation rates independently of dietary fat content in mice.

How fasting using a high fat diet still helpfully reduces dangerous cell growth.

Nutrition in 2009

PubMed ID 19084375

Effects of modified alternate-day fasting regimens on adipocyte size, triglyceride metabolism, and plasma adiponectin levels in mice.

How a 50% calorie reduction on fast days helps regulate fat cell function.

Journal of Lipid Research in 2007

PubMed ID 17607017

Physical performance and training response during Ramadan observance, with particular reference to protein metabolism.

How religious fasting creates minimal problems even in those who train or compete.

British Journal of Sports Medicine in 2012

PubMed ID 22554842

Effect of Ramadan intermittent fasting on aerobic and anaerobic performance and perception of fatigue in male elite judo athletes.

How elite athletes can even maintain high intensity physical training when fasting.

Journal of Strength & Conditioning Research in 2009

PubMed ID 19910805

Improvement in coronary heart disease risk factors during an intermittent fasting/calorie restriction regimen: Relationship to adipokine modulations.

How compared to using solid meals, Intermittent Fasting using liquid meals may be particularly protective against heart disease and be able to reduce visceral fat, faster.

Nutrition & Metabolism in 2012

PubMed ID 23113919

Ramadan fasting's effect on plasma leptin, adiponectin concentrations, and body composition in trained young men.

How religious fasting reduced body fat without interfering with appetite hormones.

International Journal of Sport Nutrition & Exercise Metabolism in 2008

PubMed ID 19164831

Modified alternate-day fasting regimens reduce cell proliferation rates to a similar extent as daily calorie restriction in mice.

How an 85% reduction on fast days causes excellent anti-cancer benefits.

Federation of American Societies for Experimental Biology Journal in 2008

PubMed ID 18184721

Dose effects of modified alternate-day fasting regimens on in vivo cell proliferation and plasma insulin-like growth factor-1 in mice.

How a 50% reduction on fast days isn't enough to get health benefits.

Journal of Applied Physiology in 2010

PubMed ID 17495119

Short-term fasting induces profound neuronal autophagy.

How fasting helps the body repair genetic errors in brain cells.

Autophagy in 2010

PubMed ID 20534972

Molecular bases of caloric restriction regulation of neuronal synaptic plasticity.

How your brain can grow new cells if you're using IF.

Molecular Neurobiology in 2008

PubMed ID 18759009

Meal size and frequency affect neuronal plasticity and vulnerability to disease: cellular and molecular mechanisms.

How your meal size and frequency affects your nervous system and brain as you age.

Journal of Neurochemistry in 2003

PubMed ID 12558961

Augmented growth hormone (GH) secretory burst frequency and amplitude mediate enhanced GH secretion during a two-day fast in normal men.

How a complete 48 hour fast causes a huge surge in growth hormone output.

The Journal of Clinical Endocrinology & Metabolism in 1992

PubMed ID 1548337

In vitro cellular adaptations of indicators of longevity in response to treatment with serum collected from humans on calorie restricted diets.

How IF can potentially increase the length of life in humans.

PLoS One in 2008

PubMed ID 18791640

Acute effects of exercise intensity on appetite in young men.

How more intense exercise is more likely to suppress appetite.

Medicine & Science in Sports & Exercise in 1988

PubMed ID 3386499

Metabolic profile of high intensity intermittent exercises.

How high intensity interval training is very effective at boosting aerobic fitness.

Medicine & Science in Sports & Exercise in 1997

PubMed ID 9139179

Impact of exercise intensity on body fatness and skeletal muscle metabolism.

How interval training, despite burning less calories during exercise, can still lead to more body fat loss.

Metabolism: Clinical & Experiment in 1994

PubMed ID 8028502

Effects of resistance vs. aerobic training combined with an 800 calorie liquid diet on lean body mass and resting metabolic rate.

How weight training helps save your muscle better than aerobic training.

Journal of the American College of Nutrition in 1999

PubMed ID 10204826

Effect of moderate-intensity exercise session on preprandial and postprandial responses of circulating ghrelin and appetite.

How walking for ages could make you really hungry.

Hormone & Metabolic Research in 2008

PubMed ID 18401836

Usefulness of routine periodic fasting to lower risk of coronary artery disease in patients undergoing coronary angiography.

How fasting improves the health of people whose heart disease requires investigation.

The American Journal of Cardiology in 2008

PubMed ID 18805103

Constitutive activation of chaperone-mediated autophagy in cells with impaired macroautophagy.

How autophagy works in your body.

Molecular Biology of the Cell in 2008

PubMed ID 18337468

Hormesis in aging.

How slightly stressing out the body can produce positive long term benefits.

Ageing Research Reviews in 2008

PubMed ID 17964227

Unexpected evidence for active brown adipose tissue in adult humans.

How scientists looking for changes in cancer tumors, discovered that humans have calorie burning BAT fat.

American Journal of Physiology, Endocrinology & Metabolism in 2007.

PubMed ID 17473055

Dietary restriction, glycolysis, hormesis and ageing.

How mice using Intermittent Fasting live longer than those using calorie restriction, which helps validate the principle of hormesis in anti-ageing.

Biogerontology in 2007

PubMed ID 16969712

Dietary factors, hormesis and health.

How mild, transient stress helps boost the body's health.

Ageing Research Reviews in 2008

PubMed ID 17913594

Nonlinear stimulation and hormesis in human aging: practical examples and action mechanisms.

How hormesis could affect a variety of health outcomes in humans.

Rejuvenation Research in 2010

PubMed ID 20662589

Comparable reduction of the visceral adipose tissue depot after a diet-induced weight loss with or without aerobic exercise in obese subjects: a 12-week randomized intervention study.

How visceral fat shrinks even without exercise, in proportion to the total weight lost by dieting.

European Journal of Endocrinology in 2009

PubMed ID 19211707

Regional fat changes induced by localized muscle endurance resistance training.

How doing weights in one area only makes the body burn fat overall, and not specifically in the exercised area itself.

Journal of Strength & Conditioning Research in 2012

PubMed ID 23222084

Resistance training is medicine: effects of strength training on health.

How weight training can prevent the muscle lost with ageing, and act like a medicine, improving a massive variety of general health improvements.

Current Sports Medicine Reports in 2012

PubMed ID 22777332

The evolution of very-low-calorie diets: an update and meta-analysis.

How very low calorie diets might not be effective by themselves.

Obesity in 2006

PubMed ID 16988070

WITHDRAWN: Advice on low-fat diets for obesity.

How the common and simplistic advice to follow a low fat diet may be incorrect.

Cochrane Database of Systematic Reviews in 2008

PubMed ID 18646093

Exercise for overweight or obesity.

How exercise works best by combining it with dietary changes.

Cochrane Database of Systematic Reviews in 2006

PubMed ID 17054187

Dietary protein - its role in satiety, energetics, weight loss and health.

How eating protein may be the most important dietary macronutrient focus.

British Journal of Nutrition in 2012

PubMed ID 23107521

Relatively high-protein or 'low-carb' energy-restricted diets for body weight loss and body weight maintenance?

How high protein in the diet could help dieters, regardless of other food intake.

Physiology & Behavior in 2012

PubMed ID 22935440

Weight-reducing diets: are there any differences?

How effective dieting may be more complex than we assume.

Nutrition Reviews in 2009

PubMed ID 19453689

Psychological interventions for overweight or obesity.

How important it is to change mentally if you want to have long-term weight loss success.

Cochrane Database of Systematic Reviews in 2005

PubMed ID 15846683

Just thinking about exercise makes me serve more food. Physical activity and calorie compensation.

How thinking about exercise could make some people overeat.

Appetite in 2011

PubMed ID 21185895

Inaccuracies in food and physical activity diaries of obese subjects: complementary evidence from doubly labeled water and co-twin assessments.

How we tend to make mistakes when remembering how much food we have eaten, and how much exercise we have done.

International Journal of Obesity in 2010

PubMed ID 20010905

Environmental factors in the development of obesity in identical twins.

How even in twins with identical genes, the effect of our behavior on body fat is clear.

International Journal of Obesity & Related Metabolic Disorders in 1999

PubMed ID 10454109

Appetite-regulating hormones from the upper gut: disrupted control of xenin and ghrelin in night workers.

How working at night could disrupt regular responses to food.

Clinical Endocrinology in 2012

PubMed ID 23199168

Is alcohol consumption a risk factor for weight gain and obesity?

How alcohol tends to increase obesity and reduce fat burning.

Critical Reviews in Clinical Laboratory Sciences in 2005

PubMed ID 16047538

Effects on cognitive performance of eating compared with omitting breakfast in elementary schoolchildren.

How skipping breakfast even in children did not affect their mental performance.

Journal of Developmental & Behavioral Pediatrics in 2012

PubMed ID 22218013

The association between alcohol consumption patterns and adherence to food consumption guidelines.

How alcohol tends to make your diet quality go down.

Alcoholism, Clinical & Experimental Research in 2011

PubMed ID 21848958

Unfavorable effects of resistance training on central arterial compliance: a randomized intervention study.

How weight training can increase the stiffness of your arteries.

Circulation in 2004

PubMed ID 15492301

The potential for high-intensity interval training to reduce cardiometabolic disease risk.

How interval training benefits your health in a variety of ways.

Sports Medicine in 2012

PubMed ID 22587821

Mere exposure to palatable food cues reduces restrained eaters' physical effort to obtain healthy food.

How just looking at food can drive you crazy when you're on a diet.

Appetite in 2012

PubMed ID 22138114

Hervey, Harris, and the parabiotic search for lipostatic signals.

How the causes of appetite are complex and not entirely understood.

Appetite in 2012

PubMed ID 22983368

Green tea polyphenols reduce body weight in rats by modulating obesity-related genes.

How green tea causes weight loss through a variety of mechanisms.

PLoS One in 2012

PubMed ID 22715380

Nutrient sensing in the gut: new roads to therapeutics?

How our guts may guide us to eat the right nutrients.

Trends in Endocrinology and Metabolism: TEM in 2012

PubMed ID 23266105

Amino acid sensing in the gastrointestinal tract.

How our guts might determine whether we've had enough protein.

Amino Acids in 2012

PubMed ID 22865248

Detecting sweet and umami tastes in the gastrointestinal tract.

How our guts might virtually taste our food and guide us to more.

Acta Physiologica in 2012

PubMed ID 21883959

Use of dietary diversity score as a proxy indicator of nutrient adequacy of rural elderly people in Sri Lanka.

How the variety of your food in your diet could be linked to general health.

BMC Research Notes in 2012

PubMed ID 22931957

Dietary diversity score is related to obesity and abdominal adiposity among Iranian female youth.

How the variety of foods in your diet could affect your level of body fat.

Public Health Nutrition in 2011

PubMed ID 20353617

Alcohol, insulin resistance and the liver-brain axis.

How alcohol could negatively affect your blood sugar control.

Journal of Gastroenterology and Hepatology in 2012

PubMed ID 22320914

Exercising for Metabolic Control: Is Timing Important?

How in healthy people, exercising on empty could be best for improving blood sugar control in the long term.

Annals of Nutrition & Metabolism in 2012

PubMed ID 23208206

Loss of autophagy in pro-opiomelanocortin neurons perturbs axon growth and causes metabolic dysregulation.

How losing a gene related to autophagy caused problems with nerve growth and also normal metabolism.

Cell Metabolism in 2012

PubMed ID 22285542

Infusion of brain-derived neurotrophic factor into the lateral ventricle of the adult rat leads to new neurons in the parenchyma of the striatum, septum, thalamus, and hypothalamus.

How adding BDNF to rats increased nervous system regeneration.

The Journal of Neuroscience in 2001

PubMed ID 11517260

Disruption of neuronal autophagy by infected microglia results in neurodegeneration.

How disruption of the normal autophagy process causes nervous system degeneration.

PLoS One in 2008

PubMed ID 18682838

The early events of Alzheimer's disease pathology: from mitochondrial dysfunction to BDNF axonal transport deficits.

How a lack of BDNF could help Alzheimer's take hold.

Neurobiology of Ageing in 2012

PubMed ID 22212405

Late-onset intermittent fasting dietary restriction as a potential intervention to retard age-associated brain function impairments in male rats.

How Intermittent Fasting later in life could still block age related brain problems.

Age (Dordrecht) in 2012

PubMed ID 21861096

Antidepressant-Like Effects of Central BDNF Administration in Mice of Antidepressant Sensitive Catalepsy (ASC) Strain.

How BDNF acts like an anti-depressant.

The Chinese Journal of Physiology in 2012

PubMed ID 23282170

Epigenetic flexibility in metabolic regulation: disease cause and prevention?

How behavior can affects our chances of being overweight and ill more than genes themselves.

Trends in Cell Biology in 2012

PubMed ID 23277089

Impact of an exercise intervention on DNA methylation in skeletal muscle from first-degree relatives of patients with type 2 diabetes.

How exercise makes a difference in those who are genetically related to people with Type 2 Diabetes.

Diabetes in 2012

PubMed ID 23028138

Fructose-induced leptin resistance exacerbates weight gain in response to subsequent high-fat feeding.

How fructose causes problems with appetite hormone Leptin.

American Journal of Physiology in 2008

PubMed ID 18703413

High-fructose corn syrup, energy intake, and appetite regulation.

How fructose in drinks tends to increase our appetite and calorie intake.

American Journal of Clinical Nutrition in 2008

PubMed ID 19064539

Dietary fructose reduces circulating insulin and leptin, attenuates postprandial suppression of ghrelin, and increases triglycerides in women.

How fructose dampens down the natural rise of ghrelin after a meal.

The Journal of Clinical Endocrinology and Metabolism in 2004

PubMed 15181085

Protein, weight management, and satiety.

How protein helps increase fullness and weight loss.

American Journal of Clinical Nutrition in 2008

PubMed ID 18469287

Dietary protein - its role in satiety, energetics, weight loss and health.

How protein saves muscles and helps weight loss.

British Journal of Nutrition in 2012

PubMed ID 23107521

IF YOU READ LEGAL STUFF

hotDNA prefers paper-free publishing wherever possible

Paperback Edition ☺ ISBN 9780957043749

STUDIO 53 • 77 BEAK STREET • LONDON • W1F 9DB • ENGLAND • INFO@HOTDNA.COM

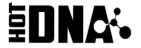

IF AT FIRST YOU DON'T SUCCEED,

TRY, TRY, AND TRY AGAIN.

– ROBERT THE BRUCE

KING OF SCOTLAND

TO HIS SOLDIERS,

THE BATTLE OF BANNOCKBURN,

JUNE 24TH, 1314.

(THEY WON)

Made in the USA
Lexington, KY
08 September 2013